T0195303

MALIGNANT

MALIGNANT

*How Bad Policy and Bad Evidence
Harm People with Cancer*

VINAYAK K. PRASAD, MD, MPH

JOHNS HOPKINS UNIVERSITY PRESS | *Baltimore*

Johns Hopkins University Press
2715 North Charles Street
Baltimore, Maryland 21218-4363
www.press.jhu.edu

Library of Congress Cataloging-in-Publication Data
Names: Prasad, Vinayak K., 1982– author.
Title: Malignant : how bad policy and bad evidence harm people with cancer
  / Vinayak K. Prasad, MD, MPH.
Description: Baltimore : Johns Hopkins University Press, 2020. | Includes
  bibliographical references and index.
Identifiers: LCCN 2019027982 | ISBN 9781421437637 (hardcover : alk. paper)
  | ISBN 9781421437644 (electronic) | ISBN 1421437635 (hardcover : alk. paper)
  | ISBN 1421437643 (electronic)
Subjects: MESH: Neoplasms—drug therapy | Antineoplastic Agents—economics
  | Biomedical Research—economics | Drug Development—economics | Health
  Policy | Patient Rights | United States
Classification: LCC RC271.C5 | NLM QZ 266 | DDC 616.99/4061—dc23
LC record available at https://lccn.loc.gov/2019027982

A catalog record for this book is available from the British Library.

*Special discounts are available for bulk purchases of this book. For more
information, please contact Special Sales at specialsales@press.jhu.edu.*

Johns Hopkins University Press uses environmentally friendly book materials,
including recycled text paper that is composed of at least 30 percent post-consumer
waste, whenever possible.

To M & A

CONTENTS

I would like to thank Sham Mailankody for his friendship and collaboration, and for encouraging me to write this book. Tito Fojo, who taught me what it means to be an oncologist. Brian Druker, Tomasz Beer, Raymond Bergan, Charles Thomas, Jeremy Cetnar, Rachel Cook, John McConnell, Sima Desai, Susan Tolle, Sharon Anderson, Tom Deloughery and many others who were advocates for my work at Oregon Health and Science University. Jennifer Gill, Alyson Haslam, David Straus, Timothy Howes, Andrae Vandross, Sally Schott, Diana Romero, Casey Zmudzinski, Diana Herrera Perez, Christopher Booth, Audrey Tran, Quiana Klossner, and three anonymous reviewers for thoughtful comments on earlier drafts of this work.

I want to thank Laura and John Arnold, Sam Mar, Meredith McPhail, and Stuart Buck for their support. Rita Redberg for her mentorship and advice. Joe Rusko for his advocacy for this book. And my many and talented collaborators whose work is featured here: Adam Cifu, Andrae Vandross, Victoria Kaestner, Derrick Tao, Matthew Abola, Emerson Chen, Bishal Gyawali, Chul Kim, Ruibin Wang, Aaron Boothby, Mauricio Burotto, Kevin De Jesus, Jonathan Edmiston, Robert Kemp, Salma Afifi, Susan Bates, Jeff Bien, Usama Bilal, Audrey Brown, Yuanbin Chen, Jessica Dreicer, Farhad Fahkrejahani, Inmaculada Hernandez, Walid Gelad, John Ioannidis, Hemnath Kumar, Austin Lammers, Eric Lu, Jia Luo, Paul Massey, Talal Hilal, Mohamad Sonbol, Christopher McCabe, Joel McLouth, Go Nishikawa, Andrew Oseran, Joseph Shatzel, Florence Shin, Kristy Duggan, and Muthiah Vaduganathan.

With love to my father, T. V. Ram Prasad, my most devoted reader.

MALIGNANT

Introduction

There is nothing so extravagant and irrational which some philosophers have not maintained for truth.
JONATHAN SWIFT

EVEN IN 2020, cancer remains a leading killer, where progress is often measured in days or weeks. Much of what makes cancer intractable is its complex and opaque biology. How does the disease originate, propagate, and, too often, dominate? Why are some cancers highly aggressive but others slow growing? Why are some parts of the body more commonly affected than others? What degree of cancer is due to genetics or inborn characteristics, and what percentage is due to the environment? What fuels the disease and how can it be hindered? What future strategies are most promising? For these questions, there are some imperfect, tentative answers based upon the best biological understanding of 2020. There are stories I could tell and references I could cite, but I will not be doing that. I will not answer or speculate about these questions in this book for the simple reason: this is not a cancer biology book.

This is a book about how the actions of human beings—our policies, our standards of evidence, and our drug regulation—incentivize the pursuit of marginal or unproven therapies at lofty and unsustainable prices. This is a book about what we can do differently to make serious and sustained progress against cancer. This is a book about how we can avoid repeating the mistakes of the past. This is a book about cancer drug policy, medical evidence, and governmental regulation. This is a book about what is entirely under our control.

There is a sad chapter in cancer history that captures many of the themes of this book. It captures how hype, money, low standards of evidence, and bias can come together to mislead cancer patients. It is a microcosm for the issues we will discuss over the course of this book. Understanding its lessons is a starting point to making sense of cancer policy. It is the story of the rise and fall of autologous stem cell transplants for breast cancer.

Stem Cell Transplant for Breast Cancer

The 1980s comprised the second decade of President Richard Nixon's war on cancer. By 1980, a number of anticancer drugs had been discovered. Most of these drugs were cytotoxic, or cell killing. They killed cells more or less proportionately to the rate at which cells undergo division. Cancer happens to have more cells undergoing division than normal cells (in many cases), and these drugs killed cancer cells preferentially. Common toxicities affected other cells that divided rapidly, such as the bone marrow (the maker of your blood cells), the lining of the mouth and intestines, and, of course, hair follicles.

Combination cytotoxic chemotherapy achieved some early successes. Diseases like Hodgkin's lymphoma and testicular cancer saw durable, long-lasting remissions, perhaps even cures. Other cancers, such as breast, colon, or lung cancer, would shrink when exposed to specific cytotoxic drugs. At the same time, impartial, empirical assessments of what had been accomplished were sobering. A 1986 article in the *New England Journal of Medicine* by John Bailar and Elaine Smith concluded that progress against cancer between 1950 and 1982 had been marginal, at best.[1]

An idea began to gain popularity. Perhaps the reason cancer drugs had not cured more tumor types was because of the insufficient dosage. If we could achieve a higher dose, we might be able to purge the body of the last, stubborn cancer cells. In a 1988 article in the *New York Times*, two expert oncologists echoed this sentiment.[2] Marc Lippman, a breast cancer oncologist, said, "It is hard to get doctors to escalate the doses of chemotherapy . . . Everyone wants to back off. But to my mind, the evidence is absolutely convincing that the dose intensity is correlated with survival." Bruce Chabner, then director of the Division of Cancer Treatment at the National Cancer Institute, said, "Doctors should raise the doses of chemotherapy 'as high as the patients can tolerate.' "

Of course, one of the major barriers to the dose of chemotherapy is the toxicity. Very high doses kill off normal hematopoietic cells—which are precursors to new blood cells—that reside in the bone marrow. Thus, an idea emerged. In order to push the dose even higher, perhaps we could remove some bone marrow stem cells, deliver a lethal dose of therapy, and then re-infuse the stem cells to save the patient. This was called autologous stem cell transplant.

During the 1980s, different groups began experimenting with this therapy, particularly for women with breast cancer. A seminal 1988 report compiled their findings. They found 172 reports of the procedure being performed. In 58% of those patients, tumors shrank 50% or more.[3] A 1992 report found that 70% of women undergoing stem cell transplant for breast cancer had tumor shrinkage, while this was true for only 39% of those undergoing conventional treatment.[4]

Tumor shrinkage, known as response rate, is a measure of tumors on x-rays or computed tomography (CT) scans, and not a measure of whether patients lived longer or better. It is a classic surrogate endpoint in oncology, that is, a measurable value that serves as a stand-in for what actually matters to patients. Moreover, these were uncontrolled experiences, so there was no direct comparison for the patients who received this experimental therapy. Ideally, a randomized trial would have been performed to test whether the stem cell transplant strategy was better than the current strategy of lower-dosed chemotherapy.

Nevertheless, newspapers promoted the idea that these transplants were better than routine care. They told anecdotes of one patient here or there who happened to do well. Experts were eager to add bold, unsubstantiated quotes to the mix. Dr. James Armitage in the *Wash-*

ington Post said, "There is a developing consensus that for some patients, this is the best available therapy."[5] Dr. Wyndham Wilson of the National Cancer Institute said in 1989, "We are now fine-tuning the procedure."[6] Of course, it is hard to fine-tune something that had not been proven in the first place. Dr. Karen Antman of Harvard said, "ABMT [autologous bone marrow transplant] can be a very effective form of treatment."[6] Again, there were no randomized trials to support this claim. The added cost of this transplant over routine care was substantial, as much as $60,000 to $200,000 at the time.[7]

Massive pressure was placed on insurers to pay for this therapy, with research of dubious value used to justify the push. For instance, a paper in the *Journal of the American Medical Association* argued that the therapy provided a "substantial benefit" and would cost $115,800 per year of life saved.[8] How was that dollar-per-life-year figure reached? By assuming that the therapy was effective in the first place.

Randomized trials were at last launched to answer the question, but they faced an uphill battle. A for-profit industry had already emerged, providing the procedure to desperate and willing women. One such firm, Response Oncology, boasted $128 million in revenue in 1998 alone.[9] Private hospitals advertised and competed for patients. A hospital owned by Cancer Treatment Centers of America even offered to pay for patients to travel to receive the treatment.[9]

In 1995, the first randomized trial found that the treatment did improve outcomes, doubling survival.[10] By 1999, that finding failed to be replicated in four other randomized trials. Eventually, evidence suggestive of fraud was uncovered for the one successful trial, and its publication was retracted. By 2000, the same physician who was so confident the key to breast cancer was just a matter of dose, wrote an editorial that served as the treatment's obituary.[11]

The failure of autologous stem cell transplant for breast cancer was not that we tried or tested the practice—it was that we applied it broadly prior to the results of well-done randomized trials. We expanded its use before we knew it worked, and we did so fueled by hype, money, hope, and bioplausibility. All together, more than 30,000 women received autologous stem cell transplants in the United States between

1989 and 1995,[12] and over 40,000 by the end of that decade.[13] This cost billions of dollars.[13] Three to 15 percent of women died during the treatment, while survivors faced massive toxicity. Patients were not helped.

I tell the (short version of the) story of autologous stem cell transplant as an introduction to this book because it is a microcosm of the themes to be covered here. It is an example of how cancer policy, not cancer biology, so often fails patients. Below are just a few of the lessons that autologous transplant for breast cancer raises and where I will discuss them further.

Many cancer therapies have astonishing and unsustainable costs. If anything, our cancer therapies have only escalated in cost since the halcyon days of the 1980s and '90s. New cancer drugs routinely cost $100,000 per year of therapy, and some more than $400,000 per dose. I discuss the crushing costs of cancer treatments and what they mean for patients and society in chapters 1, 4, and 13.

Surrogate endpoints often fail to predict which therapies improve survival. The popularity and enthusiasm for autologous transplant for breast cancer was driven by its ability to generate a high response rate. A response rate is the percentage of cancer patients whose tumors shrink 30% or more after treatment. That is an arbitrary number, and in chapters 2 and 3, I clarify how surrogate endpoints can be both effectively and ineffectively used. In chapters 9 and 11, I explain how response rate can mislead.

Randomized trials are needed in cancer medicine, and historically controlled studies often exaggerate benefit. It is difficult, if not impossible, to compare the carefully selected patients in one uncontrolled, phase 2 study against prior reports or experiences of patients, but that was the crux of the false inference regarding the efficacy of stem cell transplant for breast cancer. One hundred patients treated with this intervention did better than one hundred patients treated conventionally, but those undergoing transplant were very select people, and the comparison was flawed. In chapter 9, I discuss why randomized trials measuring survival are essential to ensuring our therapies work as well as we hope they do.

Just because something is logical or plausible does not ensure suc-

cess. It is, or at least was, highly plausible that eliminating breast cancer was a matter of dose. A wealth of basic science publications made this case, and a number of models of cancer growth and death would justify the practice. Still, just because something is plausible, even deeply plausible, there is no assurance it works. I show this lesson over and over in what follows, particularly in chapter 11.

Enthusiasts of novel therapies often hype them long before credible data are generated. Throughout this book, I show that proponents often engage in hype and that they tend not to let evidence or proof or data get in their way. The oncology drug pipeline has been called the hype-line for the way in which we let rhetoric outpace reality. Chapters 5 and 8 take a close look at hype in cancer medicine and explain why it is so corrosive.

Cost-effectiveness studies can be deeply problematic. In the case of autologous stem cell transplant for breast cancer, researchers assumed the therapy was effective and then a dollar value per year-of-life-added was calculated. However, the therapy was not effective. We assumed the very thing we should have tried to prove. We see many problems with cost-effectiveness studies in oncology, including the issue of assuming efficacy, that arise over and over. Chapters 1 and 4 describe this issue in depth.

Last, stem cell transplantation raised a slew of miscellaneous issues described in this book. Anecdotal medicine can mislead. Some patients aren't necessarily super responders to drugs or therapies but simply have slow-growing tumors destined to do well no matter what treatment is used (chapter 8). The transition between phase 2 and phase 3 trials (see glossary) is complex, and many interventions fall by the wayside (chapters 9 and 11). The role of financial and professional conflicts can be perverse (chapters 6 and 7).

In this book, I make the case that, just as with stem cell transplant for breast cancer, so much of the challenge facing cancer patients is not cancer biology but rather the inappropriate use of cancer policy. In 1999, facing difficulty in recruiting patients for a randomized trial of stem cell transplant for breast cancer, Larry Norton remarked: "Fifty years from now we will look back at this period with horror and say

'How could this have happened.' "[9] Now, 20 years later, looking back reminds us just how much our system remains the same. Bad policy and bad evidence continue to harm people who have cancer.

Audience

I wrote this book with several audiences in mind. The first includes general readers who are curious about how cancer therapies are developed, tested, assessed, priced, marketed, and discussed. The second audience includes trainees in oncology: students, residents, fellows, and even practitioners (some of us are always learning). I hope to articulate some of the implicit curriculum of cancer training, for example, how to interpret and incorporate the latest trial results in your practice. The third audience includes experts in health care policy. What systemic solutions could improve the care of people with cancer and lead to the development of more transformational drugs?

As with any book that caters to a large group of readers, I may not always be able to please everyone. Oncologists may, at times, wonder why I am repeating myself, and some topics may feel technical and abstruse for lay readers. As far as possible, I try to alert the reader to these moments and urge them to skip forward. I am hopeful that, on the whole, the themes of this book crystalize in the minds of all readers, though surely by means of diverse paths.

Controversy

Much of what I discuss in this book is controversial. I have spent considerable time providing citations and justifications for the arguments made here, and I don't expect to persuade the reader on every topic or point. I myself am open to refining or revising my thinking on any specific statement made here. Instead, I will settle for convincing you of the broad strokes of my argument:

- that more cancer clinical trials should measure outcomes that actually matter to people with cancer;

- that patients on those trials should look more like actual global citizens;
- that we need drug regulators to raise, not perpetually lower, the bar for approval;
- that we need patient advocates and experts who are nonconflicted (not receiving money from the companies who sell products to cancer patients); and
- that we must all strive to be absolutely honest in our rhetoric and free from hype.

The biology of cancer continues to unravel year by year, but, as of 2020, it remains both fascinating and opaque. There are many questions I enjoy puzzling over but know I cannot answer. The policy of cancer medicine is no less fascinating. Logical principles have emerged through practice. There is both art and science to cancer care. And, more than anything, cancer policies are human made. We created them, and insofar as the effects of those policies deviate from our goals or desires, insofar as they lead us astray, we can fix them. We can bend and break and shape cancer policy to work toward the interests of people who have cancer. Our policies can serve patients instead of companies. This book is my attempt to describe how that can be achieved.

PART I CANCER DRUGS

The Outcomes They Improve and at What Price

ONE

The Basics of Cancer Drugs

Cost, Benefit, Value

Price is what you pay, value is what you get.
WARREN BUFFETT

How Good Are Cancer Drugs?

EACH WEEK we read about new and exciting cancer drugs that are working their way through the drug discovery pipeline or have been approved for use in the United States by the Food and Drug Administration (FDA) or in Europe by the European Medicines Agency (EMA). Some of these drugs are transformative, offering major improvements in how long patients live or how they feel or function, but what is often missing from the popular narrative is that many of these new drugs have marginal or mediocre benefits. Some new drugs are even worse than this.

Let's start with one example. Imatinib (Gleevec, Novartis) is used in the treatment of chronic myeloid leukemia (CML), a cancer of the white blood cell. Full disclosure: imatinib was developed by my boss, Dr. Brian Druker, at my place of work, Oregon Health and Science University. But, ask anyone: it is a wonderfully effective drug.

In an early study where imatinib was administered to people with CML, the drug had a dramatic effect in nearly all of them. Fifty-three out of 54 (98%) patients who took imatinib achieved a complete hematologic response,[1] essentially a normalization of their blood counts. This endpoint is a surrogate endpoint—more to come on that topic—

but the percentage of patients who achieved it was astonishingly high. Many additional studies supported the use of imatinib in the years to follow—on more than surrogate endpoints—and a recent analysis shows its impact on the disease. If a 55-year-old man was diagnosed with CML in 1980, he would live, on average, an additional 3.5 years. If the same man were diagnosed in 2010, he would live, on average, an additional 27 years, which approaches normal life expectancy.[2] Some of this gain is attributable to the general trend in life expectancy—life expectancy improves for all people over time (as long as society doesn't screw up too badly)—but the majority appears to be driven by imatinib.

In contrast, most cancer drugs are not nearly this good. In an analysis of 71 drugs consecutively approved between 2002 and 2014 for solid cancers like colon or breast cancer, Fojo and colleagues found that median improvement in survival was just 2.1 months.[3] These are consecutively approved drugs, which is a fair representation of the average cancer drug that comes to market, and 2.1 months is a marginal gain. While imatinib may be transformational, the average cancer drug is not. The analysis by Fojo is not the only study of the average cancer drug. An estimate by researchers from the United Kingdom found that cancer drugs improved survival by an average of 3.4 months,[4] but this analysis likely *overestimated* the benefit.

Why do I say overestimated? First, for some drugs, there was more than one clinical trial, but the researchers chose the most favorable estimate. For instance, bevacizumab is often combined with chemotherapy for people with colon cancer. When added to a chemotherapy regimen called IFL (irinotecan, fluorouracil, and leucovorin), the drug improved survival,[5] but when added to FOLFOX (folinic acid, fluorouracil, and oxaliplatin), bevacizumab did not.[5] IFL is infrequently used in clinical practice, while FOLFOX is the mainstay of therapy. Guess which trial was selected by the investigators?

The second problem is that, in some cases where survival was not directly measured or was potentially affected by something called crossover (more to come on this in chapter 9), the authors relied on modeling studies. Modeling studies try to reconstruct or estimate what the survival would be if we could isolate the effect of the drug or follow patients long enough. The problem is that these models may be mistaken—just like a model predicting the path of a hurricane may turn out to be off the mark. In fact, the modeled estimates in this paper were consistently larger than the measured estimates.[6]

I point out these concerns not because they have great importance—frankly, there is not much of a difference between 3.4 months and 2.1 months—but to give you a flavor of what will come in this book: tips for how to better critically appraise scientific articles. In this case, whether it is 2.1 or 3.4 months, the point remains the same. Most cancer drugs are marginal, and the oncology profession owes it to people with cancer to do better.

There is an additional concern. Both the 3.4-month and 2.1-month estimates are concerned with how well cancer drugs work in clinical trials. Trials are how we assess novel drugs and are typically conducted on ideal patients—those rare people with few medical problems in excellent physical condition who have the time and commitment to participate. In the real world, cancer drugs are applied broadly to everyday Americans who are older and may have other health concerns, such as heart disease, high blood pressure, a history of stroke, or a number of limiting and disabling conditions. Marginal drugs in cancer trials wouldn't be the end of the world if the drugs were inexpensive and those small gains were maintained when the drugs were used widely. The problem is that there is mounting evidence that these gains shrink or even evaporate when the drugs are used in the real world.

Take sorafenib. In 2007, the FDA approved sorafenib to treat patients with metastatic liver cancer, or liver cancer that cannot be operated upon.[7] In the trial that led to its approval, the drug improved median survival from 7.9 to 10.7 months,[8] a difference of 2.8 months. The median age of patients in this study was 65 years old, and most had a good performance status, meaning they were active and able to take part in everyday activities.[8] In 2016, a team of researchers investigated how this drug did in the real world, using a database called SEER (Surveillance, Epidemiology, and End Results Program)-Medicare.[9] The first notable observation was that the median age of patients, regardless of whether or not they got the drug, was 70. Those receiving sorafenib in SEER-Medicare also appeared to be sicker than clinical trial patients by certain measures. People who got sorafenib were compared to a comparable group of patients who did not get sorafenib. Whether they got sorafenib or not, patients lived an average of 2 to 3 months.

Not only did sorafenib's marginal benefit evaporate in the real world setting, but the study also showed how exemplary clinical trial patients can be. The ones in the clinical trial who took placebo (sugar pills) lived an additional 7.9 months, while real world patients who took sorafenib lived less than half this time (3 months). When patients in a trial taking sugar pills live twice as long as patients taking an active cancer drug, you have an unrepresentative trial population.

How dissimilar are clinical trial patients from real world patients? Fifty nine percent of cancer patients in America are 65 years or older. And, yet, from 2007 to 2010, just 33% of people on drug approval trials were over this age.[10] Looking at patients over 70 is even more sobering. They account for 30% of Americans with cancer, but they are represented by only 10% of patients on trials leading to drug approval. In other words, trials are enriched with patients younger than most cancer patients in the United States. Others have found that trials exclude people with liver or kidney dysfunction, for instance, even if those organs are not affected by the treatments.[11] Researchers from Kaiser Permanente put this all together. They asked what percentage of Kaiser patients with lung cancer—who are broadly representative of all Americans with lung cancer—would be eligible for two randomized trials that shape treatment decisions. The answer was just 21%,[12] suggesting that trials do not enroll typical patients.

What does this all mean? Most of our cancer drugs come to market based on marginal improvements in outcomes. Before approval, these drugs are tested in patients who are healthier than the average person in the United States. When the same drugs are used in the real world—where patients are older and may have coexisting medical problems—the drug may be less effective, perhaps even approaching ineffective.[13,14]

There is evidence that these problems are getting worse over time.[15–17] Saying the situation is problematic is an understatement. If the goal of US drug regulation is to approve drugs that improve the health of Americans—and I believe this must be the purpose—then the current system is broken.

What Do Cancer Drugs Cost?

It is bad enough that most cancer drugs offer limited benefits in ideal settings and uncertain benefits in the real world, but adding insult to injury is their steep cost. In 2015, a new cancer drug was routinely priced in excess of $100,000 per year of treatment.[18] That cost bore no relationship to how well the drug worked or whether it was a novel drug (that is, operating by means of a new mechanism) versus a next-in-class/me-too drug (that is, similar to something already on the market. Think Coke and Pepsi.).[18] Globally, the high cost of cancer drugs is crushing. The cost of cancer drugs is currently in excess of $100 billion,[19] with nearly half of that spending taking place in the United States.[20]

Drug prices weren't always this high. In the 1960s, one month of cancer medicine cost $100.[21] Today, one month of a new agent is priced in excess of $10,000.[21] It is instructive to compare the growth in monthly cancer drug prices against the monthly median household income. While real wages have stagnated in the United States, the cost of cancer drugs has soared (fig. 1.1).

There is another perversity in the cancer drug market. When you have competition, the price may go up, not down. Consider imatinib. Imatinib was the first inhibitor of the protein Bcr-abl and worked wonders for people with CML. In the years that followed, multiple direct competitors emerged, such as nilotinib and dasatinib. In any functioning marketplace, the price of all three drugs would fall. Instead, the price rose. The median monthly spending on imatinib increased from $3,346 to $8,479 between the years 2000 and 2014 as it faced direct competition.[22]

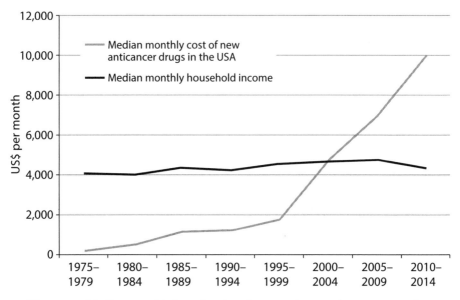

Figure 1.1. Median monthly launch price of new anticancer drugs compared to median monthly US household income from 1975 to 2014. Used with permission by *Nature Reviews Clinical Oncology.*

What Is the Value of Cancer Drugs?

We have talked about the marginal benefit of most cancer drugs. I've mentioned that these benefits are generated often under the ideal circumstances but, in the real world, results may vary. It would be one thing if these drugs were cheap, but it is quite another thing when they are so expensive. Until now, we have talked about cost and benefit separately. However, there is a term that captures both: value.

When it comes to medical interventions, one popular way to measure value is to ask: how many dollars would I have to spend to add one good, healthy year of life to the world? Health economists call this a dollar per QALY, or quality adjusted life-year. Basically, one year free of disease counts as a good year, while living with a chronic condition like cancer has a small discount. In other words, you might have to live one year and three months with cancer for it to equal living one year in good health. After all, cancer can sap your strength, make you nauseated, or cause pain. One year of living with cancer isn't quite one good year, but at the same time it is a lot better than not being around at all.

The other thing you need to know is: what is good value? Historically, health economists have believed that spending $50,000 to add a QALY is a fair price. Recent papers argue that the value should be as high as $200,000.[23] Clearly there is no right answer, and reasonable people may believe the obligations of society and the options of an individual can differ. For instance, one may believe that a billionaire should be free to pay $500,000 for one QALY, or perhaps any amount—but the same person may find it difficult to argue that society should routinely pay this much money.

Your first instinct may be shock, and your gut reaction may be "how can any number serve as a limit?" If a drug works, we should offer it, irrespective of price, the argument may go. Unfortunately, paying for costly, low-value health care involves trade-offs. For instance, money that goes toward health care is money that doesn't go toward schools, or highways, or other medical practices that may deliver far better value for money. Every dollar spent on marginal medical care has to come from somewhere else. It is a balancing act, and societies—at least rational societies—should prioritize putting money in places that deliver the most bang for its buck.

You don't have to spend too much time debating what the right cutoff for value is with cancer drugs because cancer drug value has surpassed even the most permissive thresholds. As an example: necitumumab, a drug for lung cancer, costs $800,000 per QALY;[24] regorafenib, a drug for colon cancer, costs $900,000 per QALY;[25] pertuzumab, a drug for breast cancer, costs $470,000 per QALY;[26] and bevacizumab in colon cancer costs $570,000 per QALY, which might even seem like a deal at this point, but more on bevacizumab later.[27]

These numbers are astronomically high and unsustainable for any nation in the world, even the richest. Many new cancer drugs offer poor value. Every dollar spent on regorafenib is a dollar not spent on better controlling high blood pressure. Of course, treating high blood pressure may seem unimportant when compared to treating cancer—hypertension is often silent—but the reality is that the returns (benefit to society for dollar spent) may be greater. Many years could be added to many people's lives through relatively low-cost blood pressure pills.

Nevertheless, there is an easy way to make cancer drugs a better value. We could even do it overnight if we wished. All we have to do is charge less money for them. Drug makers could lower the price of these drugs until they provided value for money and meet traditional thresholds for cost-effectiveness. The question is: how much lower could drug makers price cancer drugs and still turn a profit?

What Does It Cost to Make a Cancer Drug?

If we want to know what it costs a drug maker to make a cancer drug, there are two concepts we should review. The first is the manufacturing cost of drugs. What does it cost to make, package, and ship one pill of imatinib? The second is research and development. What does it cost to develop one cancer drug? What sort of research expenditures are needed to successfully bring a cancer drug to market?

Let's start with the first one. What does it actually cost to manufacture these drugs? Well, it depends on the form of the drug. When it comes to cancer drugs, there are two fundamental forms. The first is a small molecule. This is a chemical compound that can be made with beakers in a lab using chemical synthesis, such as Imatinib. A recent study calculated that for several small molecules used in cancer treatment, the cost to make those drugs ranged from a few hundred dollars to a few thousand dollars for a year's supply.[28]

The second common form of a cancer drug is something called a monoclonal antibody (see glossary). These tend to be larger molecules. Monoclonal antibodies are made using biology. They are like the antibodies our own bodies make and are made from cells in a petri dish or vat. Their manufacturing process is arguably more complex than that of small molecules and, for this reason, manufacturing costs have historically been higher. However, a 2009 paper takes a closer look at this. Brian Kelley found that the cost to make a monoclonal antibody can be brought down with economies of scale. In fact, it may cost as little as 1% to 5% of the sale price to make a year's supply of some antibodies.[29]

Cancer drugs cost an enormous amount of money and are manufactured for just a fraction of that price. Surely, the research and development (R&D) costs explain this discrepancy. In other words, while making an additional iPhone may be cheap, the research that went into designing the first iPhone might be quite high. For years, prevailing wisdom had been that the research and development cost for one new drug was $2.6 billion.[30] This estimate came from an analysis by the Tufts Center for the Study of Drug Development.

There are some concerns with this estimate. First, the center that conducted the research received funding from the biopharmaceutical industry. Obviously, the industry has every incentive to exaggerate the R&D cost of its products (more to come on the role of financial conflict of interest in chapters 6 and 7). Second, the analysis was nontransparent. We don't know what companies and drugs were examined and, as such, no one can externally audit the data. Third, it appears about half of the $2.6 billion figure came, not from money that companies spent, but from theoretical lost earnings on capital. What does that mean? Every time you spend $10 to develop a drug, that is $10 you didn't put in your interest-bearing savings account. A year later, the cost of that $10 is $10 plus the lost interest, which may be a few percent and the cost of inflation. In the Tufts analysis, the group used a 10.5% interest rate for the lost interest. This is a large number and a return on investment that few of us actually achieve. In this analysis, 1.2 of 2.6 billion dollars is lost interest.

Another popular analysis on this topic—from the progressive group, Public Citizen—added R&D expenses over a period of time and divided by the number of new drugs approved over this time. This method has weaknesses. First, some R&D expenses are to push products that are already approved rather than bring new products to the market. In these analyses, these dollars are counted toward developing new drugs. Second, over time, companies get larger, bloated, and inefficient, and R&D is likely no different. These analyses essentially divide the R&D

spending for future drugs, by the number of drugs developed from past R&D spending. But, R&D spending in the past was likely smaller, and the fruits of this, fewer, so this analysis may inflate the R&D to bring a drug to market. With these concerns noted, using this method, Public Citizen found that it costs $320 million to bring a drug to market.[31]

Sham Mailankody, an oncologist and researcher at Memorial Sloan Kettering Cancer Center, and I decided to update these analyses. In order to provide a transparent estimate of the R&D cost to bring a cancer drug to market, we decided to examine all of the companies that brought a single drug to market over the last decade. Using publically available securities and exchange filings, we could add their R&D expenses from the moment they began working on their target compounds.

We were able to find 10 companies that brought a single cancer drug to market. These companies had 43 compounds in human testing, only 10 of which were successful. This failure rate (77%) is broadly compatible with reported failure rates of drug development. Moreover, these companies likely had many more compounds in preclinical testing. In other ways, the companies looked representative. These companies took, on average, 7.3 years to bring a drug to market. This is consistent with previously reported ranges of 6 to 15 years. Sixty percent of drugs were approved based on surrogate endpoints, while only 40% were based on survival or quality of life. This again fits with all approved cancer drugs. Half of the drugs were novel (that is, they worked via a new mechanism of action or had a new target) and half were next in class or me-too drugs. Again, this is also consistent with all cancer drugs. At the outset, we felt our dataset was representative.

We found that it cost companies a median of $648 million to bring a drug to market. Giving credit for lost earnings on capital of 7%—a more reasonable number than 10.5% and consistent with what Warren Buffett thinks an investor can expect—our estimate rises to $757 million. This is roughly 30% of the Tufts estimate.

We took our analysis one step further. We know that cancer drugs, on average, have about 14 years of exclusivity on the market after approval, during which they can earn sizable revenue. The drugs in our analysis had been on the market approximately four years. We wanted to know what they earned in this time. Cumulatively, they earned, either through direct sales or by being acquired, $67 billion. Contrast that against the total R&D spending for all ten drugs, which was 9.1 billion. Nine of ten companies had revenues after approval greater than R&D outlays, and in time, this will surely be true for all ten. Suffice it to say, making cancer drugs is a highly lucrative business.

Is the Price of Cancer Drugs Based on Rational Factors?

The last topic worth discussing is whether the price of cancer drugs can be linked to any rational factor. If R&D outlays and manufacturing expenses don't explain the cost, perhaps cost can be explained by the benefit provided to patients. This was another question Sham Mailankody and I tried to answer. We looked at 51 consecutive drugs approved by the FDA for 63 purposes. First, we noted that drugs were approved for one of three reasons. Some drugs improved survival or quality of life, other drugs delayed the time before tumors grew past an arbitrary cutoff or what doctors call "cancer progression" (more to come on this topic), and the third group of drugs had only shown they could shrink tumors. You can think of these three categories as roughly descending order of importance. Living longer is of paramount importance, but delaying the time until tumor growth and shrinking tumors are just surrogate endpoints—or stand-in endpoints—for what patients care about.

Sham and I hypothesized that drugs that allowed patients to live longer would cost more. After all, if the pharmaceutical companies improve a meaningful endpoint, surely they would charge a premium for that. We were wrong. Drugs that shrank tumors cost the most money—approximately $160,000 for a year or course of treatment—while drugs that delayed progression or increased survival were both around $100,000 per year. Our next question was, if you just looked at drugs that delayed progression or drugs that increased survival, is there a correlation between how well the drug works and its price? In other words, if a drug extends survival by 20 months, or 500%, does it cost more than one that extends survival by 2 months, or just 10%? Amazingly, the answer was there was nearly no correlation between how well the drug worked and how much it cost.[18] You did not get more bang for your buck. In fact, for a 100,000 bucks, you got little bang.

Conclusion

Thus far, I have tried to give you the lay of the land of cancer drugs. For the most part, cancer drugs cost too much and deliver too little. Because of this, their value is poor. If you tried to explain the cost of the drugs by manufacturing prices, cost of research and development, or even the benefit they provide, you would be disappointed. In fact, the difficult conclusion is that cancer drugs simply are priced at what the market will bear. In the pages to come, I will show you that "market" is a broken, convoluted system that exerts nearly no downward force on cancer drug prices. Even calling it a market seems a stretch, but before we broach these topics, there are more basics you need to know to fully understand cancer drugs. You need to know more about the endpoints we use to approve them. Survival and quality of life are easy to master, but the surrogate endpoints of response rate, progression-free survival, time to progression, and disease-free survival are more difficult. Cancer surrogate endpoints will remind you of an onion. There are many layers. However, only by understanding surrogates, can you truly understand cancer treatment, research, and drug discovery.

TWO

Surrogate Endpoints in Cancer

What Are They and Where Are They Used?

They see only their own shadows, or the shadows of one another.
PLATO

To UNDERSTAND cancer medicine, you must have a clear idea of the surrogate endpoints used to measure the efficacy of our therapies. What is a surrogate endpoint? A *surrogate endpoint* is an intermediary, or stand-in, endpoint. It is meant to represent a clinical or patient-centered endpoint, such as living longer or having an improved quality of life, but it can be measured sooner or more easily, hence the appeal. *Clinical endpoints* are ones that inherently matter to patients, and surrogates are those that merely approximate clinical endpoints. A classic example of a surrogate is your low-density lipoprotein (LDL) cholesterol level. If you are perfectly honest, you cannot feel (in all but the rarest instances) nor do you care about your LDL but, because LDL tracks with rates of heart attack and stroke, you do worry about it. It is a surrogate for what matters. For people who suffer from diabetes, the hemoglobin A1c blood test is another example of a surrogate endpoint. It roughly correlates with the endpoints patients want to avoid, such as kidney failure, nerve damage, and blindness. Adam Cifu, a professor at the University of Chicago and my coauthor for *Ending Medical Reversal*, explains it best. Adam says, "A surrogate endpoint is something a patient didn't know was important until a doctor said it was."

Surrogate endpoints are supposed to be easier to measure than clinical endpoints, and therapy is often tailored toward improving them. For instance, blood pressure is a surrogate endpoint. It correlates with cardiovascular complications and death. We often judge the success of blood pressure medications by the extent to which they lower blood pressure. Of course, the important thing about surrogate endpoints is never to forget that they are not what you ultimately care about. They are a convenient substitute.

In this chapter, I will take you through the challenging and often confusing definitions of surrogate endpoints used in oncology. It takes a detailed understanding of how these endpoints are measured to truly understand why they are merely convenient stand-ins for how people feel or function or live, and not direct measures of those things. Much of what I discuss may be confusing. I mention statistics and graphs and percentages, concepts that may be more geared to those in the field. I encourage the reader not to get bogged down in the details and skip over confusing passages. In later parts of the book, you can refer back as needed. With this disclaimer: what are the common surrogates in oncology?

In cancer medicine, there are two major classes of surrogate endpoints: measures of tumor shrinkage and measures of tumor growth. We often call measures of tumor shrinkage *tumor response,* of which the most notable measure is the *response rate.* Tumor response means that, in a single patient, the burden of cancer has regressed beyond an arbitrary threshold. Most commonly, this is gauged using a CT scan. Take, for instance, a person with metastatic colon cancer who has several 3cm lesions in the liver, a few enlarged lymph nodes in the belly, and about 10 very small lung nodules (that have been biopsied and found to be colon cancer). We would say the patient had a complete response if all the liver and lung lesions vanish on a CT scan, and the lymph nodes return to normal size. We would say the patient had a partial response if the lesions shrank by 30% in size (the arbitrary threshold). A response rate is the percentage of patients who have complete and partial responses. If you give a drug to 100 patients similar to our hypothetical colon cancer patient and 5 have complete responses while 40 have partial responses, the response rate would be 45%.

It is worth taking a look back in history to better understand where these arbitrary cutoffs come from. Why 30% shrinkage and not 40% or 80%? In the 1970s, Moertel and Hanley invited 16 experienced oncologists to measure spheres of varying sizes through pieces of foam rubber.[1] This exercise was meant to simulate clinical practice at the time. In an era before routine CT scans, doctors had to use tools, such as calipers, to measure tumors by hand, feeling through the soft tissue, that is, the foam rubber. Moertel and Hanley asked a simple question: can you tell me which spheres are bigger and which are smaller? Of course, measuring spheres through foam rubber is not a perfect science, and two doctors could only reliably tell them apart when they were 50% smaller. From these humble beginnings, the use of arbitrary cut-points to document "response" began. In 1981, the World Health Organization established a 50% reduction in tumor area as its response cutoff. In 2000, a simplified, one-dimensional cutoff of 30% (rather than the WHO's two-dimensional measurement) was created by RECIST (Response Evaluation Criteria in Solid Tumours) and became the current standard. The take-home point here is that cutoffs that were selected for operational reasons have become codified as an oncology standard because they can be told apart with simple tools, not because they predict clinical benefit for people with cancer.

For clinical trials, there is an added complexity to response rates. If response rate is what the study is primarily designed to assess (and sadly, it often is), a researcher cannot merely document the response on a single CT scan. The researcher needs a subsequent scan to confirm the response.[2] This is done in part to ensure that the response is not simply the result of measurement error. It turns out that most measurements are done on a grainy CT scan image using a computer mouse. A flick of the wrist one way or another can inadvertently result in response if you aren't careful. With how much money is on the line with cancer drugs, one can imagine it is easy to not be careful.

From 2013 to 2015, Clovis Oncology, a pharmaceutical company, was developing a new lung cancer drug, rociletinib. Preliminary results indicated the response rate (RR)—the percentage of patients with partial or complete responses—was 59%, however, when the company confirmed the results with a second CT scan, the RR dropped to 34%. Industry experts dubbed such a change "quite extraordinary,"[3] and stressed the point that:

> for decades, a complete response (CR) or partial response (PR) in a cancer patient has required, by definition, confirmation of a defined threshold of objective tumor shrinkage by a re-evaluation performed at least 4 weeks later. Any unconfirmed responses can be reported in publications with appropriate annotations but are never the primary end point in a trial, especially in a pivotal trial designed to seek marketing authorization.

In other words, whoops!

As of 2020, the tumor burden of most cancers is most commonly assessed through radiographic imaging, and CT scans are the most common method used. Yet, depending on the type of cancer, there may be other measures of response. For instance, MRI imaging is generally the way tumors of the brain are assessed. Blood-based cancers, or hematologic malignancies, are often assessed with blood-based or bone marrow–based measurements. Circulating tumor proteins are used to gauge responses in multiple myeloma. For one blood-based cancer, CML (the leukemia I discussed in chapter 1), imatinib has pushed measuring the response even further than these other tests. The drug is so effective that amplified bits of cancer DNA are used to score response because all other measures (blood counts, etc.) are often driven to normal in nearly all patients.

The last thing to say about response rate is that it is often paired with something called duration of response. The *duration of response* is the length of time it takes for a tumor to grow more than 20% from its smallest size. The goal of cancer drug development is to have therapies that have both a very high response rate (shrink tumors for most patients) and very long duration of response (keeps them that way for a while).

Now, one might think that response doesn't sound like a surrogate at all. If a cancer shrinks, won't a patient feel better? While it is true that patients who have a response often feel better, it is not invariably the case. Moreover, there is nothing magical about 30% tumor shrinkage. Patients do not suddenly feel better at that point, and some patients may have a partial response but feel worse than when they started. Moreover, as we will see, the link between response and living longer is tenuous. Response, then, is not assurance a patient feels better, nor is it assurance a patient lives longer. Strictly speaking, it is a surrogate.

The other major category of surrogate endpoints in cancer is the time-to-event endpoints. Time-to-event endpoints are those where we measure an outcome that only happens over time. Overall survival is actually a time-to-event endpoint. The surrogate time-to-event endpoints of cancer are things like progression-free survival (PFS), disease-free survival (DFS), event-free survival (EFS), time-to-progression (TTP), and relapse-free survival (RFS). Each of these is slightly unique, and for the sake of simplicity, I will explain just the two most common.

Progression-free survival is perhaps the most common endpoint in recent cancer trials. PFS is a composite endpoint, meaning it is the time until one of several things happen. The first thing that could happen is the patient dies. This is the survival portion of the endpoint. The second thing that could happen is a patient develops a new tumor on his or her scans. The third thing that could happen is that the tumors the patient already had grown more than 20% from their smallest size. Progression-free survival is the time to one of these three events, whatever comes first, and *progression* means either new lesions on the scan or the growth of tumors more than 20%.

If it sounds confusing, it is. Progression-free survival is commonly misinterpreted in the lay press as the "time until cancer gets worse," but that isn't quite right. It is the time until a patient dies or a cancer gets *arbitrarily* worse, that is, a new lesion is seen or the tumor grows past an arbitrary threshold. It is because of the arbitrariness that it is a surrogate endpoint. Patients don't always feel their cancer progress, just as they don't always feel their cancer shrink.

Another complexity to response and progression is something I mentioned before. The percentages used to measure these outcomes, created by RECIST, are one-dimensional.[2] The 30% response and 20% progression thresholds are based on the sum of the perpendicular diameters of each mass. Why does this matter? Well, to put progression into perspective, you have to return to thinking in terms of three dimensions. The one-dimensional 20% increase in diameter dubbed progression is a 73% increase in volume.[4]

The other surrogate endpoint to understand is disease-free survival (DFS). This endpoint is also a composite, time-to-event endpoint. It is the time until either death or the recurrence of cancer. It is typically used in settings where a cancer has been fully removed and we know that only a fraction of patients will have recurrence, but we just don't know which ones. Let me give you one specific example: breast cancer. In breast cancer, DFS is a big composite endpoint, comprising several events: time to a new primary breast cancer, a new case of DCIS (ductal carcinoma in situ—a precancerous lesion), a local recurrence of breast cancer, a distant recurrence of breast cancer, or death. Not all these things are equally ominous. Death is the worst, distant recurrence the second worst, and a new case of DCIS is arguably a lesser evil.

Surrogates Are on the Rise

It is important to know about surrogate endpoints because we, in the field of oncology, are in love with them. First, the FDA loves using them as the basis for drug approval. In just six years (2009–2014), the FDA approved 83 cancer drugs, of which 31 were approved on the basis of response rate and 24 on the basis of PFS, making a total of 55 (66%) approvals on the basis of surrogate outcomes.[5] Beyond FDA drug approvals, surrogates are used widely in cancer clinical research, and their use has increased over time.

In an analysis of cancer trials over time, researchers compared the endpoint in studies between 1995 and 2004 (the early period) and between 2005 and 2009 (the later period). Overall survival (how long patients live) declined as the primary outcome, from 49% of studies to 36% of studies. Response rate was more or less stable (14% to 6%), but time-to-event endpoints like progression-free survival increased from 26% of studies to 43% of studies.[6] In short, surrogates are popular.

Surrogates Can Mislead

It is important to recognize that surrogates may fail to predict the endpoints patients care about. It is instructive to review the times these surrogates have failed to do so. In 2008, bevacizumab (Avastin) received accelerated approval (more to come on this) from the FDA for metastatic breast cancer based on one clinical trial, where its addition to chemotherapy dramatically improved PFS.[7] However, just three years later, three randomized trials failed to show that bevacizumab improved survival in the same malignancy.[8] Moreover, the benefit in PFS was smaller in these other studies than in the initial study. Because bevacizumab has harmful side effects and didn't improve survival, the FDA revoked its marketing authorization.[9]

Another example of misleading surrogates is the twisting tale of gemtuzumab ozogamicin. This drug was approved for the treatment of acute myeloid leukemia in 2000, based on an RR of 30% in a pooled analysis of three studies.[10] The drug was approved at a dose of 9 mg/m^2,* for patients older than 60 who had a relapse of cancer after initial treatment. Because the drug received accelerated approval (more to come on this topic), the company had a postmarketing commitment to show a benefit in a randomized trial. That study compared a standard treatment for leukemia with or without the addition of gemtuzumab ozogamicin at a dose of 6 mg/m^2. Unfortunately, the drug had no benefit on survival, and based on these results, the company voluntarily withdrew the drug from the market in 2010.[11,12] Then in 2017, gemtuzumab ozogamicin was again FDA approved, but this time at a lower dose (3 mg/m^2 with standard therapy or 6 mg/m^2 as a single agent). This time, a randomized trial did find a survival benefit. What's the take-home lesson of gemtuzumab ozogamicin? It reminds me of the quote by Paracelsus: "All things are poisons, for there is nothing without poisonous qualities. It is only the dose which makes a thing poison." Gemtuzumab was approved and stayed on the market for nearly a

* A milligram per square meter of body skin area is a common way to dose drugs. I could spend half a page explaining why we dose drugs this way, but it wouldn't lend greater clarity to any of the themes or lessons I wish to explore.

decade at the *wrong dose*—precisely because we embraced surrogates. Even a good drug at the wrong dose is a bad drug.

Most Surrogates in Cancer Are Poor Predictors of What We Care About

The way you judge a surrogate in cancer medicine is to ask how well it captures the change in survival. In other words, do drugs that improve response rate by 40 points improve survival more than drugs that improve response rate by just 5 points? Or, do drugs that improve PFS by eight months improve overall survival (OS) commensurately? This is called *surrogate correlation,* or *validation.*

To validate a surrogate, the process goes like this: First, you specify the cancer treatment setting you care about. Say you want to know whether cytotoxic drugs that improve progression-free survival in first-line metastatic breast cancer also improve overall survival. Here, you specify a few things: (1) the type of drug, (2) the cancer, (3) the setting (metastatic or adjuvant), and (4) the line of therapy (first or second treatment). It is important to be specific because a relationship may be strong under a specific set of circumstances but weak under others.

Second, you assemble every randomized trial that has ever been conducted under those conditions. You want to study the correlation with all of the data and not just a select group. Third, you make a graph. On one axis, you plot the change in the surrogate between the drug group and the control group, and on the other axis, you plot the change in survival. Each individual trial is one data point. In figure 2.1, I show this for a hypothetical scenario where there are two trials. In one trial, PFS increases three months and OS increases three months, and in the other it is one and one. In the figure, the change is plotted as an absolute change, but it could easily be a relative one.

Fourth, you perform linear regression, which would plot a line through the points (fig. 2.2). The tighter the points are to the line, the stronger the correlation. Every regression gives a value called the r (or *correlation coefficient*). The correlation coefficient ranges from zero (no relationship) to one (perfect relationship). The cutoffs in the figure

	Δ PFS	Δ OS
Trial 1	6.4 months – 3.4 months = 3 months	18 months – 21 months = 3 months
Trial 2	2 months – 1 month = 1 month	13 months – 12 months = 1 month

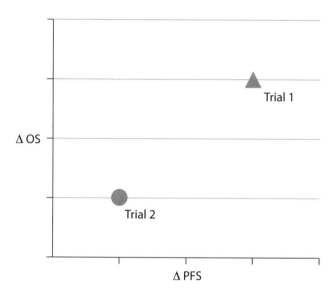

Figure 2.1. Hypothetical example of how to validate a surrogate endpoint: comparing absolute change of progression-free survival (PFS) and overall survival (OS) for hypothetical trials 1 and 2.

are those proposed by the German Group Institute for Quality and Efficiency in Healthcare (IQWiG).[13] Their proposed cutoffs are not for the correlation coefficient but the lower bound of the 95% confidence interval. This is a technical point that basically means these cut-offs are even more stringent than the numbers suggest. Some readers may think these cutoffs are quite rigid. For instance, an r of 0.7 is good. However, it is worth remembering that an r of 0.7 means roughly half of the variability in survival is not explained by the surrogate.* In the

* This requires a bit of math. We must first calculate the r-squared, or coefficient of determination.

	Δ PFS	Δ OS
Trial 1	6.4 months – 3.4 months = 3 months	18 months – 21 months = 3 months
Trial 2	2 months – 1 month = 1 month	13 months – 12 months = 1 month

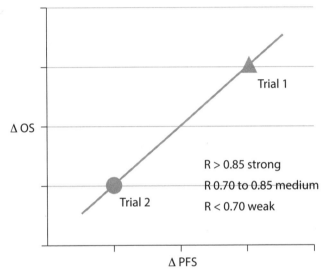

Figure 2.2. Linear regression for hypothetical example of how to validate a surrogate endpoint

real world, this essentially means large uncertainty in drugs that are approved.

In the fall of 2014, my colleagues and I decided to take stock of the surrogates we use in cancer medicine. We focused on two major settings: drugs used in the adjuvant and metastatic settings. In cancer medicine, these are the principal arenas in which we use drugs. A person who has undergone cancer surgery to remove a localized tumor will sometimes have a cancer recurrence, which may ultimately take his or her life. In the adjuvant setting, drugs are used to reduce the chance of recurrence, likely by eradicating microscopic tumor, and to improve survival. In the adjuvant setting, disease-free survival is the surrogate for survival. In the metastatic setting, in most cases (but not all), we know that no matter what we do, we cannot fully eliminate cancer. In these cases, the goal of therapy is to improve survival and quality of life, and response rate and PFS are the major surrogates.

In the adjuvant setting, we found disease-free survival was a good predictor of overall survival for lung, colon, head and neck, and gastric cancer, but not breast cancer.[14] In the metastatic setting, we examined response rate and PFS in 49 investigations. We found that 30 (61%) had poor correlations, 13 (27%) had medium correlations, and just six (12%) had strong correlations. Our review was more permissive than the German cutoffs, as we used the point estimate and not the lower bound of the confidence interval. If this doesn't make sense, don't worry. It's a minor technical point.

What about quality of life? If surrogates don't predict how long patients live, maybe they predict how well they do. Two groups examined this question. Gyawali and colleagues found, "The correlation between PFS and positive QoL [quality of life] was low (r = 0.34)."[15] And Kovic and colleagues found a "weak and nonsignificant association between PFS and HRQoL [health related quality of life]." Adding that "using PFS as the proxy for efficacy for oncology drugs is problematic."[16]

The overall conclusion is that, in metastatic cancer, surrogates are generally poor and not suitable for clinical decisions. They are better in the adjuvant setting and, to a large degree, this makes sense. Recurrence is more objective and more obvious than response and progression. Recurrence is whether the cancer comes back: either it did or it didn't. Response and progression require the measurement of tumors on scans, which, as we will see, is an imperfect art.

Surrogate Correlations Are Based on a Fragment of the Evidence

When thinking about a medical treatment, doctors are accustomed to looking at all the relevant data before drawing a conclusion. For instance, if a drug is tested in four roughly comparable randomized trials, we look at all four studies, or a pooled analysis of all four trials. The same thing is true for judging the strength of a surrogate. If there are 200 trials that measure both PFS and OS in the first-line treatment of metastatic breast cancer, we should look at the correlation between PFS and OS in all 200 trials. If you look at only a fraction of the studies, you might draw an erroneous conclusion. In the case of medical treatments, this has happened. Conclusions regarding how well Tamiflu, a widely used and stockpiled antiflu drug, works depend strongly on how many studies you look at and whether you consider both published and unpublished trials.[17,18] The more unpublished studies you examine, the more it appears Tamiflu is a marginal or useless drug.

My colleagues and I previously examined the breadth of articles included in surrogate validation meta-analyses studies.[14] We found that no analysis looked at all the relevant trial data. Only 14% (5/36) of analyses searched for unpublished trials. Unpublished studies are vitally important to include, as these can change conclusions regarding medical treatments and are often unpublished for a reason—their findings, though factual, may not be what the community wants to hear. In the case of surrogates, unpublished trials may have different relationships than those that are published.

We took a close look at the five articles that surveyed the unpublished literature. They identified 684 trials they wanted to include in their study, but they could not access data needed from nearly half the trials. They went forward with 51.5% (352/684 trials) of the data they had identified as relevant. You don't have to be an expert to know that one should take any conclusion with a grain of salt if it is based on only half the pertinent data. The same is true for surrogate validation studies. I personally would love to see a complete analysis.

Do Surrogates Speed Up Approvals?

I introduced the surrogate as an endpoint that is measured before survival, so naturally it would seem logical that using surrogates would speed drugs to market. In 2018, Emerson Chen, Sunil Joshi, and I attempted to estimate the time saved by accepting surrogate endpoints.

Adjusting for the line of therapy, a measure of disease severity, and the speed with which a trial can accrue, a measure of both desirability of the study and prevalence of the condition, we found that surrogates speed drugs to market by 12% over only accepting overall survival. In other words, if drug development routinely takes 7.3 years, a move to overall survival would increase time to 8.2 years.[19]

But, maybe the truth is a bit more complicated. Here is a tricky idea to grasp, but is it possible that using surrogates doesn't speed new drugs to market? Imagine we lived in a world where surrogates were not accepted. If you were a drug company, there would be only one rational place to study drugs: among cancer patients whose tumors had grown despite using all conventional therapies. This group of patients is unfortunately at the highest risk of death from cancer, and if your new drug works, it will show a benefit very quickly in this group. As a general rule of statistics, the ability for a successful drug to show it is superior to an alternative gets higher as the risk of a bad outcome goes up. In patients who have exhausted other options, the risk is as high as it gets.

Now imagine we live in a world that accepts surrogates. What happens now? You might think that companies, the prime architects of clinical trials, will run the same trial they otherwise would, but using the surrogate. That might happen. Then again, the company might see a different opportunity. Instead of going after patients who have failed other options, what if the company were to go after people with a new diagnosis of the cancer, who have not tried any drugs? If you were assessing overall survival, it might take a while, but a surrogate might be faster. Moreover, if the drug does work, think about the market share. Instead of getting a *third-line* (people alive and well after two prior courses of therapy) market, you would get a *first-line* (or *front-line*) market, which includes many more patients/consumers.

It just might happen that the surrogate in the front line and survival in a later line would take approximately the same amount of time to reach. Thus we can imagine, hypothetically, a company deciding to use the surrogate for bigger market share, instead of speed. Has this ever happened?

Consider the situation of two different HER2-directed therapies in metastatic breast cancer (TDM-1 and pertuzumab). One was approved in the *second line* based on overall survival, the other in the front line based on progression-free survival. The funny thing is that the time from when these trials started enrolling patients to the moment the results were finalized was very similar (42 and 40 months, respectively).[20] It certainly looks like speed was traded for larger market share with pertuzumab. Of course, this example does not prove that drug companies adjust their behavior this way, but I think the important lesson is to keep one's mind open. The acceptance of surrogates may have unintended consequences. In fact, that is true for many things in life.

Conclusion

This chapter lays the groundwork for understanding the surrogate endpoints we use in cancer medicine. Both response rate and progression-free survival have to do with cancer shrinking or growing *past an arbitrary threshold*. Because this threshold was selected arbitrarily, it should not be surprising that, as a general rule, these endpoints fail to predict overall survival or quality of life. Moreover, their widespread acceptance may have the unintended consequence of encouraging manufacturers to conduct trials in earlier disease settings, bartering speed for market share. In the next chapter, I dive deeper into surrogate endpoints and ask how they are used for regulatory decisions and whether that makes sense.

THREE

The Use and Misuse of Surrogate Endpoints for Drug Approvals

Statistics are no substitute for judgment.
HENRY CLAY

D RUG REGULATORS have embraced surrogate endpoints. The FDA
approves two-thirds of cancer drugs on the basis of an improvement in surrogate endpoints such as response rate or progression-free
survival.[1] The European Medicines Agency approves a similar percentage of cancer drugs based on surrogates.[2] The last chapter provided an
introduction to the surrogate endpoints used in oncology, and some of
their weaknesses. Here, we focus on how drug regulators use these
endpoints to usher promising and not-so-promising compounds to the
clinic.

In the US market, there are two types of regulatory approvals that
the FDA can give companies. The first is *regular approval*. With regular approval, the FDA has largely declared itself satisfied with the efficacy of a drug and tends only to ask for further safety information.
The second is *accelerated approval*. Accelerated approval is sometimes
referred to as provisional approval. With this stamp, the FDA essentially says that, while it thinks the drug is promising, the company
must have a future commitment to prove the drug improves a clinical
endpoint, such as survival, once it is on the market.

Accelerated approval is the ideal process for dealing with surrogates.
It strikes a balance by making a drug available sooner while completing
a validation trial later. Regular approval is ideal for drugs that have

already shown survival or quality-of-life benefit. Yet, surrogates are used for both types of approval, and this is where things start to get messy.

If you review regulatory language for accelerated approval, you'll find that the FDA is obliged to use a surrogate that is "reasonably likely to predict."[3] That kind of language is vague, and reasonable people may disagree just how strong a surrogate validation study needs to be to demonstrate it is "reasonably likely to predict." For regular approvals, the language states that a drug must improve survival, quality of life, or an "established surrogate."[4] Here, I think reasonable people might find more agreement. An established surrogate must be a surrogate with a fairly strong ability to predict survival. In fact, the FDA uses cut-offs for the correlation coefficient similar to the ones discussed in the last chapter to define established surrogates.

In 2016, Chul Kim and I decided to explore these issues.[5] We looked at all FDA cancer drug approvals over a six-year period and found 83 approvals. First, we confirmed that 66% (55/83) were based on a surrogate endpoint. Next, we noted that 25 of the 55 surrogate approvals were accelerated approvals and 30 were regular approvals. Surrogates were used for all accelerated approvals and more than half of regular approvals.

Every time a surrogate endpoint was used to approve a cancer drug, we performed a systematic review of the literature to find a study documenting the strength of the correlation. We figured reasonable people can disagree about how strong is strong enough, but no rational person would defend the absence of having studied the question. We found for 14 out of 25 accelerated approvals (56%) and 11 out of 30 regular approvals (37%) there was nothing. No, not a study showing a poor correlation. I mean nothing. Either no one had ever looked at it or, if they had, they didn't think it was worth publishing. Moreover, I think it is unlikely that the FDA has studied these endpoints and not published those results, partly because when the FDA does study surrogates, it seems eager to publish its findings, even if those findings are weak.[6,7] Our results were concerning. They imply that many surrogates are based on little more than a gut feeling. You might rationalize that and argue a gut feeling is the same as "reasonably likely to predict," but no reasonable person could think a gut feeling means established. Our result suggests the FDA is using surrogate endpoints far beyond what may be fair or reasonable.

Let's also examine what happened when we were able to find a published correlation. Previously, I talked about the r cutoffs for surrogates. For accelerated approvals, we could find four approvals (16%) where there were surrogate validation studies reported the r. All four were low correlation ($r \leq 0.7$). For regular approvals using surrogate endpoints, 15 approvals (50%) had a study capable of giving us the r value. Three (20%) had high correlation ($r \geq 0.85$) with overall survival, four (27%) had medium correlation ($r > 0.7$ to $r < 0.85$), and eight (53%) reported low correlation ($r \leq 0.7$). So, when proper studies were done, they mostly showed weak correlation between the surrogate endpoint and overall survival. Again, while you might rationalize a weak correlation as "reasonably likely to predict," I think it is a stretch to call it "established."

The FDA Fails on the Back End

Despite this tough take on surrogate endpoints, I personally believe some cancer drugs should be able to be approved based on surrogates. For cancers with few treatment options and poor outcomes, I believe drugs can be made available based on surrogates as long as future studies assess overall survival and quality of life and they report the results after approval. If these studies are negative, then the drug should be pulled from the market; if positive, then patients and doctors benefit from more accurate estimates of benefit. This thinking is in line with the original philosophy of accelerated approval. However, as we will see, the FDA uses surrogates for new drug approvals in excess of this—many times for cancers that already have established, effective treatment (more to come).

Here, however, I wish to focus on the back end of drug approvals. Even if the FDA is lax with granting approvals up front, it wouldn't be the end of the world if it was strict on the back end. As long as it enforced postmarketing commitments and made sure surrogate approvals actually led to patient-centered benefits, I think we would survive. Unfortunately, the FDA fails to do this. The first way it fails is by giving regular approval for surrogates. This essentially waives the need to perform postmarketing commitments. The second way it fails is by not enforcing the postmarketing commitments made through accelerated approval.

Consider the first reason: granting regular approvals based on surrogates. In the previous chapter, I discussed bevacizumab in breast cancer. It was approved based on PFS and revoked when it failed to show a survival benefit. In 2012, the FDA approved everolimus in breast cancer.[8] This drug was like bevacizumab, in that it was used in addition to usual therapy and approved based on a PFS improvement. There was one difference. It got regular approval instead of accelerated approval. For this reason, when the long-term results of the drug's trial failed to show a survival benefit, the drug was not revoked by the FDA, and it remains on the market.[9] To get the full picture of the concerning efficacy data, serious toxicity, and extensiveness of everolimus's effect on patients with cancer, I recommend reading the 2015 expose published by the *Milwaukee Journal Sentinel*.[10]

Now the second reason: failing to enforce postmarketing commitments. In a 2017 study by Steven Woloshin and colleagues,[11] the authors examined 614 postmarketing studies that were promised to the FDA. Five to six years after the promise was made, 20% of the studies were never started, 25% were ongoing or delayed, and 54% were completed. The FDA could impose fines on the responsible companies but has never chosen to do so. These results echo a 2009 report from the Government Accountability Office (GAO), which also found the FDA was lax in its enforcement of postmarketing requirements.[12]

What does this mean for cancer drugs? In 2015, Chul Kim and I decided to find out. We took every drug approved that was based on a surrogate and asked: with an average of 4.5 years of follow-up, how many showed survival benefit? The answer was just 5/36, or 14% of postmarketing studies. This percentage showing survival benefit was 1/15 accelerated approvals (7%) and 4/21 regular approvals (19%).[1] A few years later, a study of approvals by the European Medicines Agency found similar results.[2] Whether cancer drugs must show survival or quality of life gains *before* approval is debatable, but no sensible person can think they should *never* show these gains. Since so many drugs are marginal and cost so much, the current regulatory standard appears inadequate.

"Unmet Medical Need" and the FDA Drug Approval Process

To better understand how regulators use surrogate endpoints, we have to learn more about the phrase "unmet medical need." In chapter 5, I explore the use of language in cancer therapy and how often it can be inappropriate, exaggerated, or misleading. Now is the time for a sneak preview. "Unmet medical need" refers to a condition for which there is no adequate method for prevention, diagnosis, or treatment. The phrase "unmet medical need" is among the most overused phrases in cancer medicine. Each year, we see researchers labeling cancer settings as unmet needs, even when there have been a flurry of new drugs approved for those conditions. Why are we enthusiastic about this phrase? It turns out if you call a cancer an "unmet medical need," it empowers the FDA to use the accelerated approval pathway for that cancer setting.[13] And, guess what? Everyone wants to use that pathway.

In 2017, my colleagues and I examined the use of "unmet medical need."[14] We found that the phrase was used to label a spectrum of cancers: cancers that were rare with no treatment options and poor five-year survival, as well as cancers that were common with dozens of treatment options and a rather good five-year survival. I think it is fair to say that a common cancer setting with many treatment options and a favorable survival is not as "unmet" as a rare disease with few options and poor outcomes. And yet, we found this phrase was used indiscriminately. Is it possible that the phrase "unmet medical need" is overused in cancer medicine precisely because it permits the option of accelerated approval, which facilitates the use of surrogate endpoints for approval? That was the hypothesis we were left with, and one that I think is highly plausible.

By the Time You Validate a Surrogate, Is It Too Late?

In 2017, I worked with Robert Kemp, a medical student from the United Kingdom. Robert made the observation that surrogates don't save that much time, if you think about it. Why? His logic went this way: we ought to be reluctant to use surrogates that are not validated because they may be erroneous. For this reason, we should wait until they are validated to use them. However, before one can validate a surrogate, one needs many trials that measure both the surrogate and the hard endpoints in a specific setting. As a simple matter of fact, it may take years to build that knowledge base. If a new class of agents comes out, we will be unsure whether our surrogates work equally well. It is a bit of a catch-22: by the time you establish your surrogate, you may not need it after all. His conclusion: it might be better to stick with clinical endpoints.

Why Are Response Rate and PFS Deficient?

Part of the reason why response rate and PFS are not reliable surrogates has to do with how they are measured. Although measuring the size of cancer sounds like it should be straightforward, it isn't. It is less like measuring your height and more like measuring the width of a cloud. The border is often ill defined and hazy. Where does one cloud end and another begin? This is akin to measuring tumors on a scan.

There is a wealth of data to support the idea that the variability in tumor measurements over time and across readers can lead to misestimates of response and progression. In a meta-analysis of all published studies examining the agreement between two observers, Yoon and colleagues found that there was marked disagreement when the same scans were scored by different readers or the same reader at different time points. In many cases, a response (shrinkage of tumor of 30%) or progression (growth of more than 20%) could occur simply by variability in tumor measurement.[15]

In a single study, where the same scans were given to multiple radiologists and oncologists who scored responses or progression events, the response rates ranged from 4.1% to 20%, depending on who did the scoring.[16] Progression occurred in as few as 8% of patients or as many as 29%, again depending on who measured the scans. The key thing to remember here is that these were the same exact images.

Censoring

Measuring response rate and progression offers more problems than measurement error. We may not be considering the right denominator of patients. In 2017, the FDA approved the first cellular cancer therapy, called tisagenlecleucel (Kymriah, Novartis), or CAR-T, for short. A CAR-T is a chimeric antigen receptor T-cell, basically a genetically modified cell taken from a patient that is trained to attack cancer cells and then placed back in the patient. In the data submitted to the FDA, 88 patients had the cells removed, but 18% (16/88) did not receive the cells because some patients died and some patients' cells could not be manufactured.[17]

Unfortunately, the FDA excluded these patients from the denominator and assessed response only in patients who got the cells. This violates a principle called *intention to treat,* that is, you should judge a drug based on all patients allocated to get it, irrespective of whether or not they received it. Why? Because therapies that take a long time to give (this CAR-T took approximately 22 days to make) may exclude the sickest patients who die while waiting, thus distorting their benefit. In fact, if I have a patient in my office and we decide to treat with tisagenlecleucel, the response rate from the package overestimates her chances of success, as I am unsure she will live long enough to receive the cells. With progression-free survival, however, there is an additional form of selection bias.

Progression-free survival is a time-to-event endpoint. That means that we care about the time until something happens. In this case, we care about whether the time-to-progression or death is, on average, longer in one group of patients than another. When you sit back and look at the data for a time-to-event endpoint, you will notice a few things. Some people had the endpoint or event. Some people did not. Of those who do not have the endpoint, there will be a range of follow-up. For instance, one person may have been watched for a year without having the event happen, whereas another person may experience the event after just two months. Some patients who did not experience the endpoint may have been lost to follow-up, but the outcome is unknown.

With modern clinical trials, if the endpoint is overall survival, it is rare that a patient is lost to follow-up. After all, investigators can simply call the patient or her family and find out she passed away or is still alive and doing well. Progression-free survival is a different story. To document progression, a patient has to continue to return for follow-up visits and undergo CT scans. Clinical trials often mandate that CT scans be done at set time points, such as every six or eight weeks. These time points are often far more frequent than real-world clinical practice.

Additionally, if patients decide to stop returning to their appointments or seek care elsewhere, they become "censored." Censoring means that we remove these persons both from the numerator and the denominator. We don't assume they progressed. Rather, we simply assume they are missing and instead weigh a bit more heavily the patients who did return.

Imagine a drug that has substantial toxicity. If this drug has side effects so bad that people give up taking it, some of those patients may also decide to stop returning to the clinic for the specified scans. After all, why go see a doctor whose treatment you are no longer taking? If this were to happen, these patients would be censored and data for these patients would be weighed less than others. One of the big assumptions of time-to-event analysis is that the patients who are censored are no different from those who return. In other words, they are not healthier, wealthier, or wiser. But, if the people who drop out experience a disproportionate amount of side effects, it is possible they are also having those side effects because their bodies have less reserve due to more advanced cancer. In other words, frailer patients may be the ones more likely to stop the drug.

What does this mean? Putting it all together, we might have something called *differential and informative censoring*. Differential, meaning patients are more likely to drop out of the study if they were assigned the study drug (and not placebo) because the drug has toxicity; and informative, meaning the patients who drop out are different from those who remain (maybe they have worse cancer or are sicker). In such cases, if we throw out the data of the sickest patients and weigh the remaining ones, we likely overestimate how good a drug is and may even create false inferences about the drug's efficacy.

Has this ever happened? It is hard to prove that it did. Yet, a recent trial called BOLERO-2 raises suspicions. In this study, patients were randomized to an antihormonal drug with or without everolimus, a drug mentioned earlier in this chapter. Everolimus is one of the toxic, marginally beneficial, costly new cancer drugs we have discussed before, and was profiled in the *Milwaukee Journal Sentinel*. In this trial, many patients were censored very early on in the study, and it appears (from visual inspection) that this happened at a higher percentage in the everolimus arm.

In 2014, I spent a year at Johns Hopkins University. At that time, I met Usama Bilal, an epidemiologist. Usama wrote a computer program to reconstruct the progression-free survival in the BOLERO-2 trial, assuming patients who were censored were more or less likely to have progression than those who remained behind.[18] In other words, Usama made six curves for this trial, seen in figure 3.1. Patients getting everolimus are in light gray, and those getting placebo are in dark gray. The thick solid lines are the reported results and the dotted lines and the thin solid lines are the results assuming patients who were censored all lived, or all died.

By altering the assumptions about what happened to the censored patients (whether or not they had immediate progression or never had progression), we could get the curves to cross. Essentially this means that the observed PFS benefit could be explained by differences in the patients who were censored.

To be clear, our analysis does not prove that censoring sick patients created the benefit seen in BOLERO-2, it merely suggests that the benefit seen could evaporate if one made different assumptions regarding the censored patients. It provides another reason why PFS gains do not

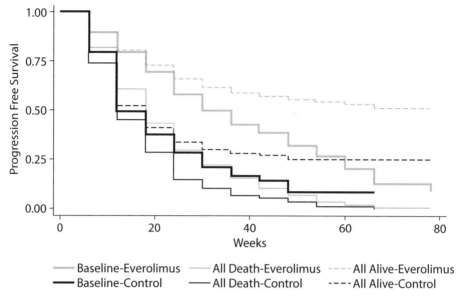

Legend		
── Baseline-Everolimus	── All Death-Everolimus	---- All Alive-Everolimus
── Baseline-Control	── All Death-Control	---- All Alive-Control

Figure 3.1. The role of censoring in BOLERO-2. Best-case and worst-case scenarios for censoring in the BOLERO-2 study. Thick, solid lines represent actual progression-free survival (PFS) curves reported from trial. Dotted curves represent PFS if every censored patient had no progression. Thin, solid curves represent PFS if all censored patients experienced progression. Used with permission by Elsevier *European Journal of Cancer.*

always yield OS gains. PFS can be distorted by loss to follow up in a way survival cannot.

Surrogate Threshold Effects

The last topic to broach is something called surrogate threshold effects. Basically, there are some people who agree with the argument here. Yes, it may be the case that changes in PFS are a poor predictor of changes in OS. However, this does not mean PFS is useless. What if a four- or six- or ten-month improvement in PFS could provide assurance of an OS benefit? In other words, is there a magnitude of PFS benefit after which it does predict overall survival?

There are two things here worth pointing out. First, the simple fact is few drugs have large PFS gains. Consider the article by Fojo and colleagues,[19] which found, among 71 consecutively approved drugs, a median improvement in PFS of 2.5 months, with only 3/71 drugs (4.2%) offering more than six-month gains in PFS.

Second, asking if there is a "threshold" above which PFS becomes reliable introduces a thorny problem, which I will discuss more in chapter 9. It is called the problem of multiplicity. *Multiplicity* means that the more chances you have to achieve something, the more likely, by chance alone, you will get an outcome you desire. For instance, if someone wants to gauge how good you are at shooting a basketball, they might give you 10 or 20 shots and take your average. But what if they allowed you take a thousand shots, and only present a videotape of the best 10? Given a chance like this, anyone can be José Calderón.* Surrogate threshold makes this problem a reality because you could conceivably draw the threshold at any one of infinitely many locations. For instance, you could ask if a 4-month, 5-month, 6-month or 6.2-month threshold predicts overall survival, and infinitely many more cutoff values.

In a threshold analysis, as long as there is any positive trend between a surrogate and survival, and there very well might be, then one will be able to draw a line somewhere to find a "useful" cut point. Even a weak, fleeting, and unreliable correlation may have some favorable cutoff. But this is hardly trustworthy. Whether we can operationalize surrogate threshold effect is the subject of future research, and it still may fall victim to the problem outlined by Robert Kemp.

What Do the Regulators Have to Say?

The claims presented here are concerning. Most new drugs come to market based on unreliable or untested surrogates. They appear to utilize regulatory pathways (for example, regular approval) in violation of stated standards (that is, for surrogate endpoints that are not established). It would be one thing if drugs came to market with ongoing trials meant to resolve uncertainty, which seems acceptable, but unfor-

---

* Highest free throw percentage in an NBA season

tunately, we don't test them rigorously on the back end. As a result, many cancer drugs stay on the market for years without proof that they improve outcomes patients care about. This situation is troubling.

For a long time, we could only speculate about what regulators thought about these problems. Then, one of them decided to explain himself. Writing in the *BMJ*, Francesco Pignatti, Head of Oncology, Haematology and Diagnostics at the European Medicines Agency, addressed these thoughts.[2]

First, Dr. Pignatti argued that it is difficult, if not impossible, for cancer drugs to show survival benefit when a patient uses several drugs in succession. Whatever gains may happen as a result of the first drug are "diluted" by subsequent drugs. In other words, the drugs patients use after they finish the trial can dilute the benefit of the tested medication. There is a formal term for this argument. It is called the "survival post protocol" argument.[20] When survival after the new drug is long, the benefit of the drug could be diluted, the argument goes.

A picture is worth a thousand words in characterizing this argument. In figure 3.2, each arrow is a drug. Dr. Pignatti, and many others, argues that the new drug (arrow) didn't show improved survival because its benefit was diluted by the subsequent old drugs (arrows).

But step back and think about this. If a new costly cancer drug is really so beneficial, the survival benefit *should not be able to be matched* by all the older, inferior drugs. If you could achieve the same survival with all the old drugs we have, what precisely does the new drug add?

An analogy may help. Imagine you are running a marathon. Normally, you drink Gatorade to keep you going without leg cramps. Now, someone sells you a special energy drink that can only be drunk once at mile marker 2. Imagine you run miles 3 and 4 slightly faster than you otherwise would, but you lose steam and run miles 18 and 19 slightly slower than you normally would have run them, even though you go back to using Gatorade for these miles. In the end, you finish at the same time. Would you conclude that the value of the drink was diluted by the subsequent miles or that the new drink adds nothing?

The second argument Dr. Pignatti makes is that conducting studies to measure survival or quality of life become impossible for drugs with

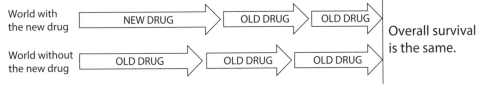

World with the new drug: NEW DRUG → OLD DRUG → OLD DRUG

World without the new drug: OLD DRUG → OLD DRUG → OLD DRUG

Overall survival is the same.

Figure 3.2. Visual of the "survival post-protocol" argument. The argument claims that the positive effects of new treatments (arrow) are diluted by older, subsequent treatments (arrows), making it difficult to judge a new drug's benefit. But, if how long you live is the same, then what value did the new medicine truly provide?

high response rates. After all, if most patients have tumor shrinkage, shouldn't they also have better quality or longer length of life? Unfortunately, this is a twisted view of these surrogates. If a high response rate were a guarantee of survival or quality-of-life benefit, then we would accept response rate as a reliable outcome, but the fact is, it isn't. There are drugs that show huge response rates (>60%) that have failed in randomized trials assessing survival and have been pulled from the market.[21] Another problem with this claim is that the response rate in early trials is frequently inflated. They are bigger than rates seen in subsequent testing. In a famous comparison of 49 early trials against 43 follow-up randomized studies using the same drugs for the same cancers, 81% of the response rates were larger in the early studies.[22] If high response rates prevent randomized trials, one can never learn the true response rate, or whether drugs truly help people. The final problem is that among drugs approved based on response rate, the outcomes are generally unexceptional. In another paper I worked on and led by Emerson Chen,[23] we found that, among drugs approved based on response rate, the median response rate was 41%, and the median complete response rate was just over 6%. That is a far cry from imatinib with its 98% complete response rate (chapter 1), and rather modest.

Dr. Pignatti's final point is claiming the world is better off with surrogate approvals than without it. This, however, is speculation. We don't know what a world without surrogates would look like. While Dr. Pignatti fears that eliminating surrogate endpoints would needlessly delay drug access, the reality could be quite different. Drug companies may learn that they cannot pursue drugs that merely improve surrogates. They may retool their entire R&D portfolio to chase better drugs. The world might be better off if overall survival was the default endpoint for approval. Of course, I don't know if this is true, but one can speculate in either direction.

Conclusion

In this chapter, we finish our tour of surrogate endpoints in cancer medicine. Regulators heavily utilize them, and academics are eager to label many conditions "unmet needs," facilitating the use of more surrogates. This might be acceptable if we later held these drugs to a higher standard, but too often the FDA fails on the back end, and thus, drugs remain on the market for years, and neither patients nor doctors know whether or to what extent they improve survival or quality of life. Arguments used by regulators as to why the status quo cannot be reformed seem to be lacking, and a more rational use of surrogates seems to be an easy way in which we can improve cancer drug policy.

Terminology

A final note on nomenclature. Thus far, I have introduced a lot of terms. I have defined *adjuvant* and *metastatic, progression-free survival,* and *response rate,* but there are a few terms you need to understand, and this seems to be the best point at which to explain. Let me tackle a few basics here, and for a more detailed list, please see the glossary.

Cancer drugs have different mechanisms of action. The major categories of these mechanisms are cytotoxic therapy, targeted therapy, immunotherapy, and cellular therapy.

Cytotoxic drugs are chemotherapy agents that preferentially kill dividing cells. They tend to kill cancer solely because these cells divide more quickly than normal cells. Their side effects often target hair, gastrointestinal tracts, and bone marrow because these cells undergo more division than other healthy cells. Chemotherapy alone can cure several cancers—testicular and lymphoma, for instance—and increase cure rates after surgery for many others—lung, breast, and colon, for example.

Targeted drugs are both small molecules and antibodies (recall chapter 1) that are directed against specific cancer proteins or molecules.

Immunotherapy drugs are those that utilize the body's immune system to attack cancer. There are several classes: (1) Cancer therapeutic vaccines are vaccines given to people who already have cancer to encourage their own body to attack the tumor. With one exception (discussed in chapter 9), cancer therapeutic vaccines have universally failed in testing. (2) Cancer checkpoint inhibitors are a blockbuster class of medications that make it more difficult for cancer to escape the body's immune system, and they are often described as "unleashing" the immune system. (3) Cellular therapy are cells made outside of the body and re-infused in order to attack cancer. The most notable version in recent years is called CAR-T. Finally, (4) bone marrow transplants from one person to another, which have existed for decades, are a form of immunotherapy.

The last bit of nomenclature worth knowing is the line of therapy. If a patient presents with metastatic cancer and received a series of treatments, changing when the tumor progresses, each agent in the series is called: first line, second line, third line, and so on. Subsequent lines refer to second and beyond. Relapsed or refractory refer to tumors that return after a period of absence or do not appear to shrink in response to therapy, respectively, as a general rule.

[FOUR]

How High Prices Harm Patients and Society

For what is worth in anything
But so much money as 't will bring?
SAMUEL BUTLER

IN CHAPTER I, I explored the high cost of cancer drugs, a problem that is crushing patients, their families, and society. The topic of the cost of cancer drugs is too vast for just one pass, so let's take a closer look at some of what we missed: Which drugs are rising in price? What does it cost to bring a drug to market? And how do we judge the value of a new drug?

Which Drugs Are Rising in Price?

The launch price of cancer drugs when they debut has been steadily increasing from a few hundred dollars for a one-month supply in the 1970s to $10,000 for a one-month supply today.[1] The problem of high cancer drug prices applies to more than just the newest medications. To understand this, however, we need to take a quick detour into infectious disease.

In the fall of 2015, Martin Shkreli and Turing Pharmaceuticals achieved notoriety for taking a treatment for an infectious disease related to HIV, pyrimethamine, and jacking the price way up. What was once $13.50 a pill was now $750 a pill. Of course, pyrimethamine is generic and sold for about 5 to 10 cents in other nations. In the months that followed, it became clear that the business model for some com-in the pharmaceutical drug sector was to take advantage of older drugs that, for many reasons (including historical accident), were being made by a single supplier.[2]

The case of Turing Pharmaceuticals and other high-profile cases raised the question: Did this also happen in oncology? Which drugs undergo the largest price increases, new or old ones?

To test this hypothesis, my colleagues and I downloaded publicly available data from Medicare Part B, which comprises drugs that are administered in physicians' offices or hospitals. We selected all drugs that were available in both 2010 and 2015, so a newly approved drug in 2012 would not be included. We adjusted prices for inflation and then asked how much the price for each drug changed between 2010 and 2015.

We found a few things. First, some drugs had a marked reduction in price over these five years.[3] That reduction tended to happen when multiple (not just one) generic manufacturers came on the scene. Second, a few drugs had astonishing price increases. One had more than a 1,000% increase in price. It wasn't the new drugs, however, that had the biggest price increases. It was the old drugs (fig. 4.1). In other words, the strategy of taking older drugs and raising their price is not just seen in a few exceptional cases, but part of a broader pattern.

What Does It Cost to Bring a Drug to Market?

In the first chapter, I summarized a project my colleagues and I completed on the R&D costs of bringing a drug to market. We found that it costs $757 million to bring a cancer drug to market. We arrived at this figure by picking companies over the prior 15 years that brought one cancer drug to market, and then we added up their spending on all successful and unsuccessful compounds.

These companies got 10 drugs approved out of 43 that were in clinical trials—a success rate of 23%. This success rate is identical to the 26% reported by DiMasi and colleagues from the Tufts Medical Center in the *Journal of Clinical Oncology* (see fig. 4 in DiMasi et al.).[4] In other words, our portfolio of companies appeared to fail at the same rate documented by prior analyses.

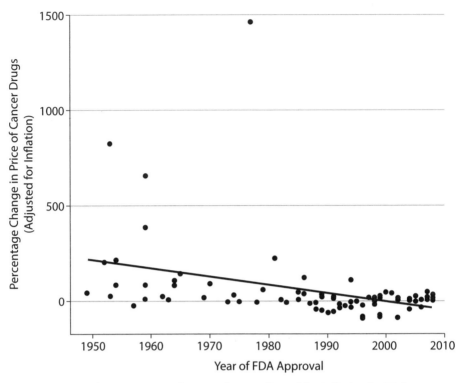

Figure 4.1. Change in price of cancer drugs, adjusted for inflation by FDA approval date (in percentages). Used with permission by *JAMA Oncology*.

In the weeks that followed our analysis, there was some criticism. One argument was that we only looked at winners. Where was all the R&D spending for companies that flopped? We believe that it doesn't make sense to include those companies. If you want to know what it costs to put a man on the moon, it would be sufficient to add the entire NASA budget of the 1960s. Would you add the space budget of Belize and China? If you include every company that fails, and expect drugs prices to pay off all of their outlays, you are asking that investment into the biopharmaceutical sector become risk-free.

Another argument was that we focused on small companies and not large ones. This was an inherent limitation of our method, which involved studying companies that brought their *first* drug to market. However, there is a reason not to study large companies. Many of the trials run by large companies, which constitute R&D expenditures, may not be R&D in the way one might conceive of it.

Consider a recent paper by Mattina and colleagues.[5] These authors studied the entire published development plan of a single cancer drug, sorafenib. They found the drug was approved after two trials testing its efficacy. What followed was testing in 26 different cancer settings and in 67 combinations, leading to just one additional approval. There were 3,928 patient-years (this is basically just multiplying patients by the number of months they were on study and then dividing by 12) swallowed up by all of the sorafenib trials. This tells us that the R&D for sorafenib took a lot of patients' time. What is most damning is that only 93 patient-years, or 2% of the time, were spent on the first approval and the rest was spent on all the other, mostly low-value, testing.

What does this have to do with the cost of R&D? It means that if you look at big companies' expenditures, some of what they spend on R&D is to bring the drug to market, but probably much more is spent trying to get a second use for the drug patients already have. Because these companies are large and have enjoyed large and steady profits, they may be inefficient.

The bottom line about the varied and diverse estimates of pharmaceutical R&D is that there is no need for estimates because we can actually measure it if we choose to. Transparency in drug companies' accounting, which may come through legislation, could easily answer this question. Normally, I would say such a proposal is too intrusive, but because drug companies use the cost of R&D as a justification for high drug prices, one may argue that it would be fair and reasonable to explain just how expensive R&D is.

Cost-Effectiveness Research

As discussed in chapter 1, there is one metric that is incredibly useful to compare the value of different medical practices, even practices that seem very dissimilar (for example, surgery, preventive medicine, and a drug used to treat cancer). It's called the dollar-per–quality adjusted life-year, or QALY. Although there is debate about just how much society should be willing to spend for new medical treatments, some experts argue that the threshold should be as high as $150,000 or $200,000 per QALY.[6] I discussed how some cancer drugs are far beyond this. They have QALYs that approach a million dollars! This is an absurd figure that no rational society can continue to pay.

In 2015, researchers from Tufts University looked at all the cost-effectiveness studies of drugs for blood-based cancers in their own dataset and found that the majority looked like a good deal.[7] Eighty-six percent of these drugs had value ratios of less than $100k per QALY, and 73% were less than $50k. This figure was surprising. Sure, some cancer drugs for blood-based tumors may be good deals, but 73% of them having less than $50k/QALY? That seemed too good to be true. My colleagues and I took a close look, and we found five things that were problematic and wrote a rebuttal in the journal *Blood,* a colorfully named and prestigious medical journal.[8]

First, we noted that the authors didn't look at the cost-effectiveness of all drugs for hematologic malignancies (blood-based cancers) over the time span they examined (years 2007–2012). They didn't even look at a random set of drugs. They looked at 29 studies of nine drugs that just happened to be in their database. At the outset, this raises the concern that the articles included are not a representative or random sample, but rather a sample skewed toward favorable conclusions.

Second, 22 of the 29 studies were funded by the industry. That doesn't just look fishy, there are data that show it is fishy. A review of industry versus non-industry-funded cost-effectiveness studies found that when the industry pays for the study, it is roughly three times more likely to find that a drug is less than either $50k per QALY or $100k per QALY.[9] In other words, not only does Tufts use a *convenience sample*—a term for things it happened to have on hand, which could introduce bias—its sample is steeped in industry studies, which are known to be favorable toward cost-effective results.

Third, some of the studies were conducted using costs of health care from nations besides the United States, and then final costs were back calculated into US dollars. I cannot stress how problematic this method is. Unless you have been asleep for the last 20 years, you will agree that everything in the US health care marketplace is distorted and US prices are far different from global prices. To know what the value of a drug is in the United States, you can't crunch the numbers in rupees and then back calculate.

Fourth is the big one—a problem I often harp on—some of these cost-effectiveness analyses assumed the effectiveness part. In other words, some of these studies measured surrogate endpoints but modeled/projected/imagined what benefits these drugs might have on the endpoints that matter—survival and quality of life. Take one example used by the Tufts researchers. In one analysis, the authors estimate the value of continuing rituximab, a newer drug for patients with relapsed follicular lymphoma. The analysis postulated that there would be a 12-percentage point increase in survival at five years, from 61% to 73%. Yet, when updated data from the trial were finally reported, there was no survival benefit at all. So the entire dollar-per-QALY calculation is essentially null and void. Yet, this was included among the successes of the Tufts study.

I want to take a minute to expand on this point. Before you conduct a cost-effectiveness analysis, you have to know that a therapy is effective. You have to prove someone lives longer or better as a result of a therapy. You cannot take a response rate and turn it into quality of life. You cannot assume a longer PFS is the same as living longer. When you assume efficacy and use those numbers in your value calculation, you are essentially making things up. We learned this lesson with autologous stem cell transplant for breast cancer in the introduction. This is not to say that you cannot make any assumptions when you conduct a cost-effectiveness analysis. The nature of the method ensures that you have to make assumptions. But, one of those assumptions should not be the very notion that the intervention works because that is the prerequisite to even doing the analysis.

Years ago, I pointed out the irony that you can find cost-effectiveness analyses saying that some medical practices are a good deal, only to find later those practices are ineffective, or worse, what I call *medical reversals*.[10] A medical reversal is a medical practice that is widely embraced and adopted and years later found to be no better or worse than a prior or lesser standard of care.* In order not to look foolish, it is a good idea to perform a cost-effectiveness analysis if, and only if, the efficacy of the therapy (that is, the fact it works) is actually known.

The fifth and final rebuttal to the Tufts paper is the simple fact that when you look objectively, systematically, and comprehensively at cancer drugs, the value tends not to be good. Howard and colleagues[11] looked at 58 consecutive drug approvals for which survival was measured or modeled (okay, I really don't like the modeled part but, if anything, that should make the analysis look more favorable). They found only 34% of approvals had values less than $100k per QALY. Looking at 14 drugs for blood-based cancers in their dataset, 43% came in less than $100k per QALY and 29% less than $50k per QALY. So instead of 86% and 73%, you get 43% and 29%—that is a sizable difference. Moreover, I suspect that if you were a little more of a methodological purist and excluded modeled benefits, the differences would be even more sobering.

There is a sixth concern about cancer cost-effectiveness studies, which my colleagues and I did not cover in *Blood,* but is worth knowing about. Whenever cost-effectiveness is calculated, it is always incremental. That means, compared to doing X, it costs this much more to add a year of life to do this new thing, Y. The problem is that when the Xs begin to cost more and more, the Ys, in comparison, don't look so bad. If you are slightly cheaper and equally effective or ineffective, or slightly more effective and only a tiny bit higher in price than an already outrageously priced drug, then you start to look really good.[12] In other words, a Ferrari clearly costs more than a Honda, but compared to a Bentley, it doesn't look so bad.

Why spend so much time talking about cost-effectiveness studies? Because it is imperative to understand that they are malleable. They bend and fold like a piece of tin, and the person who runs them can manipulate them, evidenced by the aforementioned fact that industry-sponsored studies are three times more likely to reach positive conclu-

---

* If you are interested in this topic, you should read my first book, *Ending Medical Reversal,* which I wrote with Dr. Adam Cifu, professor of medicine at the University of Chicago.

sions. The devil is in the details. Did the therapy prove survival benefit, or are we merely guessing it might have one? Did the authors use US dollar figures or Russian rubles? Are they comparing the new drug to an older, cheaper one or an equally pricey, and not so old therapy (a misleading comparison)? There are far more layers and nuances to cost-effectiveness than I have described here, but I hope this is illustrative in showing why we cannot just accept values that get bandied about without verification.

CAR-T

There is one specific medical therapy that is worth revisiting because it captures many of the emerging challenges when it comes to cost, efficacy, and value of cancer drugs. That drug is a "living therapy" and is the chimeric antigen receptor T-cell, or CAR-T for short.[13] I briefly discussed it in chapter 3 regarding response rates.

A CAR-T is a cell from a cancer patient that has been engineered to attack a particular target, ideally something expressed in abundance on the surface of a cancer cell. It's made in a stepwise fashion. First, a cancer patient's cells are removed from his or her body intravenously. Those cells are sent to a laboratory, where the T-cells (a type of infection-fighting cell) are isolated. T-cells need two signals (called co-stimulation) in order to attack, a general warning signal and infection-specific signal. A piece of DNA is shoved into the patient's extracted T-cells to activate the danger signal and tell the cells to produce a receptor against a specific target (cancer cells). The cells with this added DNA are grown until there are enough cells to ship back to the doctor and patient.

The patient gets a preparatory dose of chemotherapy and then the cells are infused. This chemotherapy is intended to allow the body to receive the modified cells without attacking them, but it is possible that these drugs exert some direct anticancer effect. What happens next can be a rollercoaster ride. Many patients can develop illnesses like sepsis, that is, a really bad infection. Neurologic problems are emerging as a potential toxicity of the medication as well. Some patients develop low blood counts that do not improve for months.[14] A few fortunate patients are left with very low levels of cancer cells, and some may even have total clearance of the cancer.

To date, CAR-T cells have been approved for pediatric acute lymphoblastic leukemia (ALL) and adult non-Hodgkin's lymphoma, though it is not hard to imagine that, even as you read this, more approvals have been given, mostly for blood-based cancers (would be my guess). This rudimentary understanding of how CAR-T works is necessary to think about the policy implications, of which there are several key concerns.

First, how well does the drug work? Let's take axi-cel (axicabtagene ciloleucel), which was approved for relapsed, refractory diffuse large B-cell lymphoma. The drug was tested in 111 patients, but I am going to scale everything as if it were a 100 people, in order to make the numbers easy to think about.

If 100 people went to the doctor and had cells collected, 91 would be able to get the manufactured product (with that DNA bit inserted). Nine people would either be given the bad news that their product could not be made; die in the 17 days, on average, it takes to make the cells; or get too sick to get the cells. Eighty-two people will have tumor shrinkage. Of these, 44 will still be in remission six months later. For a few reasons, it is impossible to know how these patients would have fared with conventional therapies.

First, such a comparison would be a *historically controlled study,* and, as I show in chapter 9, those are notoriously unreliable and prone to overestimate benefit. Second, in this case, it would be particularly difficult to compare these patients with historical controls. By the time this study was enrolling, it was widely known that CAR-T was highly promising, but the therapy itself could take patients to hell and back with its side effects. Many clinical centers reported long wait lists. If you have a wait list, and open up spots at random, you essentially select for indolent biology or, in other words, patients whose tumors are naturally growing slowly. An analogy may help. Imagine you go to a busy restaurant on a Friday night. The host takes your name on a waitlist but makes no promise how long it will take. As spots open, the host goes down the list to find someone who is still there to take the table.

You can imagine that on average, people who leave the restaurant—fed up by the wait—are probably hungrier than the ones who patiently wait for their name to be called. Similarly, if you have a waitlist for patients with a terminal malignancy, those with more aggressive tumors tend to die while waiting, and those with slow-growing cancers are more likely to hear their name called.

Additionally, knowing the toxicity was formidable, doctors likely relied upon their judgment to decide if a patient was well suited or fit enough for the therapy. For these two reasons, CAR-T studies were likely composed of patients who were healthier, on average, and more likely to do better no matter what treatment they got, making comparisons to historical data unreliable.

Consider the numbers for the other CAR-T approval, tisa (tisagenlecleucel), which was approved for pediatric and young adult relapsed refractory ALL (a type of leukemia). With tisa,[15,16] of 100 people who get cells collected, 81 actually get the modified cells. An unlucky 19 either die or have a manufacturing failure, meaning the cells cannot be made. Sixty-seven people will respond to the cells—CR (complete response) or CRi (complete response and incomplete recovery of blood cells). Of the responders, just 43 will still be in remission at one year.[17] Again, comparing this to the alternative is impossible, but the point I want to make is that, in both cases, the majority of patients, 56% to 57%, will not benefit in the long term from this new product. It is probably fair to call CAR-T good, fair to call it a step forward. But, we must not forget that the majority of people who desire the therapy will relapse or die, and that, frankly, is not good enough.

Now, let's talk about the price. Tisa costs $475,000 for the one-time dose, but there has been talk about some small discount. Axi-cel costs $373,000 per dose. These are astronomically high prices, but by asking a few questions, we can see that there are a few reasons why the situation is even worse than it seems.

How much of the development of CAR-T was funded by the US federal government? A patient advocacy group called Patients for Affordable Drugs, led by David Mitchell, a cancer patient himself, added up all of the government grants for CAR-T and found the total was $200 million. Compare this to the estimate of what Kite Pharmaceuticals (developers of axi-cel) spent. In *Nature Reviews Clinical Oncology*, I added the R&D from public Securities and Exchange filings for all available years at the time (2012–2016) and found the total was $304 million.[18] Thus, the cost of bringing the drug to market was a blend of public and private funding. If anything, the public funding was offered during the most vulnerable period, when no one knew whether CAR-T would succeed or fail. The private funding occurred only when the prospect of commercialization seemed large.

How much does it cost the companies to make the cells? Carl June, the developer of the tisa CAR-T, told the *New York Times* that it cost his lab $20,000 to make the cells.[19] Moreover, this admission occurred back when the cells were being made the hard way, in a small laboratory, when costs were highest. One would imagine that magnitudes of scale would lower—not raise—the manufacturing price. Since Kite, the maker of axi-cel, was acquired by Gilead for $11.9 billion, the company has already reaped tremendous revenue and will likely continue to make out handsomely for years to come.

Is $475,000 the entire price? It turns out that the price of these medications is just the base price. Giving CAR-T requires collection and infusion costs, and there will be the costs of managing the frequent side effects, which can include lengthy hospitalizations. Through some quirk of fate, a costly rheumatoid arthritis drug became the standard way to treat the worst side effects of CAR-T, and the price of this medication will have to be shouldered by patients and payers. My colleagues and I estimated that the increased costs of ancillary treatments could rise to the tens of thousands of dollars.[20] Finally, given that these drugs have the rate of relapse that I described above, some providers may be dissatisfied with using CAR-T alone. For the young people with leukemia, doctors may want to follow CAR-T with a bone marrow transplant, which will add another few hundred thousand in costs. In short, the price of the cells is just the tip of the iceberg with CAR-T. There are a lot more therapies coming down the pipeline, including some gene therapies, which may cost as much as or more than this.

Conclusion

Here we delved deeper into some of the intricacies and challenges of the cost of cancer drugs. As with CAR-T, unless you understand how the therapies work and how effective they are, you cannot understand if the prices are fair. Reasonable people will agree that we need profits to serve as an incentive to develop drugs, but there is a difference between profits that motivate and profiteering. Moreover, as with CAR-T, the federal government—taxpayers—often shoulder a significant burden of funding high-risk science. For this reason, it would seem evident that there should be some checks in the system to ensure equitable prices, fair profits, and a fair distribution of profit to those who bore the greatest risk, which in many cases are the US taxpayers.

PART II SOCIETAL FORCES THAT DISTORT CANCER MEDICINE

FIVE

Hype, Spin, and the Unbridled Enthusiasm That Distorts Cancer Medicine

Oft expectation fails, and most oft there
Where most it promises.
SHAKESPEARE

WE HAVE covered several important topics to frame the way you should think about the treatment of cancer, but this survey would be incomplete without discussing the social, political, and cultural forces that affect cancer medicine. In part II, I hope to show how prevalent hype and financial conflicts of interest are in cancer medicine. Understanding the nature of these forces will help us make sense of some of the challenges I outlined in part I and some of the problems with cancer clinical trials I will describe in part III. In this chapter, I tackle the pervasive issue of hype.

If you Google the term *hype*, you will find this: "extravagant or intensive publicity or promotion."* When it comes to cancer drugs, we are drowning in hype. Every new drug seems to be a miracle, breakthrough, game changer, or cure, irrespective of how well it works or for how many people. Journalists, investors, and doctors seem to be having a secret competition to see who can serve the largest superlative salad about every new therapy.

Consider one drug: palbociclib. Palbociclib is added to hormonal therapy in metastatic breast cancer and is approved based on an im-

---

* https://www.lexico.com/en/definition/hype. When I grew up, I kept a tattered, paperback dictionary on my nightstand, and it was a trusted companion. But times have changed.

provement in progression-free survival. The drug was first approved by the FDA in February of 2015. As of this writing, the drug has not shown an overall survival benefit—the outcome that actually matters to patients—in any single study to date. In fact, palbociclib is a lot like bevacizumab in breast cancer—a drug that improves a surrogate (PFS) at the price of toxicity and cost ($12,000 per month).[1] Yet, that doesn't stop newspapers from running headlines hailing the drug as a game changer. Examples of this are: "Hope for Breast Cancer Patients as 'Game Changing' New Treatment Could Delay Gruelling Chemotherapy for Months";[2] " 'Game-Changing' Breast Cancer Treatment Delays Growth of Tumour";[3] and "Breast Cancer 'Game Changer' Hits New Zealand—but Only for Women Who Can Afford It. Despite Being Fast-Tracked by the FDA in the United States, Patients and Charities are Hoping Ibrance [Palbociclib] Can Receive Public Funding."[4]

Game changer is a loaded term but one that is subjective. In my mind, a game changer is a drug that transforms outcomes for patients. Imatinib was a game changer, and we should be working to find drugs as good as imatinib. Instead, some wish to lower the bar and use *game changer* indiscriminately. I believe there are some clear hallmarks of a game changer drug that are missing in many hyped drugs today. What do game changer drugs look like?

While it is clear that response rate is a surrogate endpoint and does not guarantee patient benefit, drugs with low response rates have nearly no chance of meaningfully improving survival. Most cancer drugs have response rates below 50%, for instance. In order to even entertain the language of *game changer,* I think you should have a response rate in excess of 50%. How can a drug be a game changer if the majority of people don't even experience tumor shrinkage? Once we clear this hurdle, we must ensure that responses last a very long time. Finally, and most important, the therapy has to change survival outcomes for the disease. It must make patients feel better. A game changer should ideally restore the life expectancy of the majority of patients who take the drug to normal, as imatinib did (chapter 1).

A good rule of thumb for a *game changer* is this: a game changer is the kind of drug where, if the doctor had the disease, he or she would breathe a sigh of relief. That's true for HIV drugs. That's true for imatinib. That isn't true for palbociclib or bevacizumab.

Game Changers, Miracles, Revolutions, Cures, and Home Runs

Game changer isn't the only word I often hear. Alongside it, I find *revolution, miracle, breakthrough, unprecedented,* and *cure. Unprecedented* has an incontrovertible meaning, and in a short while, I will give you objective data on its use. *Cure* is also a very specific term that we have studied formally. *Revolution, miracle, breakthrough*—are all subjective terms. Their meaning is in the eye of the beholder. Nevertheless, there must be some legitimate boundaries to their use.

In 2015, I attended the annual cancer meeting in Chicago. Like most meetings, this was drizzled in superlatives. I heard all the terms already mentioned, as well as *groundbreaking, lifesaver, marvel,* and *home run.*

Matt Abola and I decided to formally study superlatives. We made a list of 10 superlatives and searched news.google.com to identify when they were used to describe a cancer drug. Matt quickly had a stack of 94 articles that used superlatives. The use of superlatives came from a broad collection of news outlets—66 by our count. Among those 94 articles, 97 superlatives were used, referring to 36 specific drugs. Our research questions were simple: who was using superlatives and what drugs were they praising?

Our results were published in *JAMA Oncology.*[5] We found that half of the drugs (18 of 36) that received superlative mentions had not received FDA approval. More concerning, we found that 14% (5 of 36) had never been given to a human being. These drugs had only been given to mice or tested on cancer cells in a petri dish. Any cancer researcher knows that the odds of a drug that works on mice or in a test tube also helping a human being are low—perhaps as low as winning the lottery. To celebrate these drugs in the lay media seemed irresponsible.

Who was using superlatives? Well, it was mostly the journalists and/or authors of the news stories (55%), followed by physicians (27%), industry experts (9%), patients (8%), and a member of congress (1%). Among the classes of medications called superlatives, 38% were immunotherapy drugs like nivolumab and pembrolizumab.

Five percent of superlative use was for describing a therapeutic cancer vaccine. First described in chapter 3, therapeutic cancer vaccines have had high rates of failure among all cancer therapies. There has only been one ever approved by the FDA, and there are a number of concerns regarding its approval (see chapter 9).

Unprecedented Results?

What about a word with an incontrovertible meaning? Something like *unprecedented*? Lexico.com defines *unprecedented* as "never done or known before." For simplicity's sake, let's agree that an unprecedented drug is one that is better than anything that ever came before in that cancer. Each year, I hear researchers using the word at our national meeting to describe new drugs. In 2016, my colleagues and I decided to put this to the test: were unprecedented drugs truly better than prior medications?

We used Google News and Medscape (a physician website) to identify cancer drugs whose benefit was hailed as unprecedented, and then identified something called the *hazard ratio* for either overall survival or progression-free survival (depending on what data are being referred to). A hazard ratio is roughly a measure of the difference between a drug and placebo across time. A hazard ratio of 0.8 is like saying the risk of the bad outcome (either death or progression or both) is 80% as likely, or 20% less likely, at any point in time if you get the drug. When it comes to explaining cancer medicines to patients, a hazard ratio is not very useful, as it tells you nothing about what a patient might actually expect.[6] It doesn't tell you the likelihood of a bad event happening. It could be 100% likely to happen in a year, or one in a million, and a drug can still have a hazard ratio of 0.8 but, for the purposes of testing whether a benefit was truly unprecedented, it is useful. It is a single number that can be compared against all prior drugs and trials to see how much better than a prior standard of care a new drug is (proportionately), and that is precisely what we set out to do.

We found 96 instances of *unprecedented* being used, and we made a few observations. First, researchers were most likely to use the word (59%), followed by journalists (38%), CEOs of pharma companies (2%), and one from a practicing doctor. In these 96 instances, *unprecedented* was stated to describe 48 drugs used to treat specific cancers. Only 52% of these drugs were FDA approved for that particular cancer, and 4% had been tested only in animals or the laboratory (you already know what I think of that). For 26 drugs, we were able to find a randomized trial documenting the benefit on either survival or progression-free survival. Now, here was the kicker. In 23% of these examples—roughly one in four—we were able to find a prior study with a superior hazard ratio. In other words, we could prove this drug was not unprecedented. It had a precedent. We had already seen something better.

Putting it all together, we found that only 40% of the time has an unprecedented drug been tested in a randomized trial where no better drug could be found. We conclude in our paper, "the use of the word 'unprecedented' in the lay press is often inaccurate and frequently overstates the importance of findings from the scientific literature."[7]

Use of the Word *Cure* in the Scientific Literature

It isn't just articles in the lay press that use glowing terms inappropriately; it also plagues biomedical literature. Biomedical articles are those that appear in scientific journals that form the currency of academics and are a measure (appropriate or inappropriate) of one's success.

In 2014, I performed an empirical analysis of how authors use the word *cure* in papers appearing in the biomedical literature. I searched Web of Science for all 2012 articles that used *cure* in their title under the category of oncology. I was able to find 29 full articles that used the word *cure* in the title, referring to one cancer or another. Again, these were not articles in the lay press. These were academic articles in biomedical literature. The stuff careers are made of.

I wanted to know: how many articles used *cure* correctly? To do that, I had to answer one question first: What's the correct meaning? In 1963, Easson and Russell put forth a wonderful definition of *cure* that we haven't improved upon, in my opinion. They said a cure occurs when, after some treatment has finished, a patient has the same chance of living a long and full life as a person of the same age and sex who never had the disease.[8] In other words, the survival function returns to that of healthy people.

If you think about it, this definition captures what we mean by *cure*. A cure is a fixed course of treatment that results in your health being restored. Your chance of living a full life should be the same as if you didn't have the disease. At once, you might see the problem with cancer treatments. Some cancer therapies have side effects or toxicities that might compromise your chance of a full life. You may be rid of the problem that faces you, but years may be shaved off your life expectancy. This situation would fall short of cure, as Easson and Russell saw it.

Therefore, I wanted to know, of the 29 articles that used the word *cure* in the title, how many authors used it in a way consistent with the Easson and Russell definition. The answer was just 10, or roughly one in three. I also wanted to know how many authors used *cure* to describe a situation in cancer medicine that was presently (as of 2014, when I did the study) considered incurable. The answer was that 48% of the time *cure* was used to describe an incurable situation. These findings reminded me of the lines by Alexander Pope:

Hope springs eternal in the human breast
Man never is, but always to be blest.[9]

Which, in my mind (and here I am no expert) means that humans have a tremendous capacity for hope. Yet, we are never satisfied with what we have, and always want another blessing.

Predicting the Future

The last term I want to talk about is the phrase *inflection point*. Recently, I have noticed that national leaders use this term to mean that we are on the verge of seeing faster cancer breakthroughs—we are at the inflection point. Scott Gottlieb, the former commissioner of the FDA uses this language. Gottlieb states, "I think we've finally reached an inflection point in science where we have the techniques sufficiently perfected to actually allow these products to be translated into therapies for humans."[10] José Baselga, the former physician in chief of Memorial Sloan Kettering Cancer Center, also employed the word. Baselga says, "We have indeed reached an inflection point, where the number of discoveries that are being made at such an accelerated pace are saving lives and bringing enormous hope for cancer patients, even those with advanced disease."[11]

These experts contend we are on the verge of faster breakthroughs. But, of course, there is no way to know that. Moreover, the history of oncology is replete with experts believing that we are on the cusp of a major breakthrough. For example, in a 1998 *New York Times* story, James Watson was quoted about fellow researcher Judah Folkman, "Judah is going to cure cancer in two years."[12] Two years later, cancer was not cured. In 2003, Andrew Von Eschenbach, head of the National Cancer Institute, outlined a proposal to "eliminate suffering and death" from cancer by 2015.[13] This promise did not materialize. To his credit, Von Essenbach later told reporters that statement "was the biggest mistake of his life."[14] Suffice it to say that the history of cancer has not validated the soothsayers who spoke of impending cures.

Time for Spin

Hype is often employed in situations when you don't know the results of a study or the future of a field, or for embellishing positive results. But, what can happen if we already have negative results? The answer is something called *spin*. Spin is a type of bias, a way to distract readers from negative results.

A famous paper by Vera-Badillo and colleagues explored spin.[15] Researchers looked at 164 randomized trials of breast cancer published between 1995 and 2011. Fifty-six percent were negative for the primary endpoint, which is roughly comparable to all randomized trials in cancer. The primary endpoint of the study is a study's raison d'etre. It is the reason the trial was done and typically the only endpoint the trial has the power and scope on which to comment. Vera-Badillo found that 59% of the negative trials reached for some other finding, any other finding (typically a secondary endpoint), to try to portray the experimental therapy favorably. This was spin—pure and simple.

In a subsequent study, some of the same researchers pushed this concept. They took 30 papers with spin in the abstract—the short summary at the beginning of a paper that generally is the only part of a paper people read. They rewrote all 30 without spin. Then they randomized 300 docs to read the abstract with or without spin. They found that readers thought the interventions in abstracts with spin were more likely to be beneficial and were more likely to want to read the whole paper.[16]

It reminded me of a long-standing observation of mine about excessive flattery. Even though it seems obvious to a third party that someone is kissing up, the person receiving the flattery often buys it. Even though these abstracts clearly play up negative findings, doctors are more likely to see the upside and want to hear more. It confirms a nagging suspicion that I have had for years: doctors are people too and susceptible to the psychological forces that govern us all.

Medicine by Press Release

Recently, on Twitter, a colleague asked if any doctors were going to embrace the results of a new randomized trial called ECHELON-1.[17] This trial tested whether substituting a new and costly drug for a tried and true older drug improved outcomes in Hodgkin's lymphoma. While a surrogate endpoint—modified progression-free survival*— was improved, overall survival was not reported. Will we change practice because of these results? I was still thinking about it when an as-

---

* Since the writing of this chapter, the trial has been published, and many experts, myself included, have been skeptical whether the results should change practice. For instance, see http://www.ascopost.com/issues/january-25–2018/echelon-1-a-commendable -study-but-questions-remain/.

tute oncologist remarked, "Ask us once we've seen data, not press releases."[18]

That was exactly right. Ask us when we have read the paper, seen the data, and gotten more facts than a threadbare press release. Yet, cancer treatment and research seems to be moving in the other direction. In 2013, for instance, a press release came out about concerning negative trial results that lenalidomide increased death in chronic lymphocytic leukemia,[19] but the paper didn't come out until nearly four years later.[20]

Allowing press releases to drive medicine permits fragments of information to guide the narrative and prevents others from taking a close and critical look at information. In fact, it is probably fair to say a press release is the antithesis of how science should be disseminated.

Meetings

No discussion of hype would be complete without identifying the most common source of hype: professional academic conferences. These are lavish, opulent affairs held in grand convention centers and too often doused with industry funding. At the major national oncology conference, ASCO, held annually in Chicago, attendees have to walk through industry booths on the way to the posters. The pharmaceutical displays are commanding and grandiose. I used to joke that you could twist your ankle in the plush carpeting of the displays—it was that luxurious.

Do medical conferences have any value? Presumably, they have two goals: to disseminate findings as rapidly as science happens, and to meet and network. Yet, mounting evidence suggests that the first goal may be distorted or perverted, perhaps leaving us with only the latter.[21]

Consider the fact that many presentations at conferences are abstracts. In other words, short snapshots of a research study and its findings. These are typically so short that not enough information is included in order to make an educated assessment of them. I can tell you the number of times I have read an abstract and felt, "That is persuasive. I will start doing that and don't need to read anymore." The answer is never.

By now, it should not be surprising that findings presented at conferences may have spin or hype, but here I want to focus on the disconnect between these findings and subsequent publication. At the outset, let me say that even published papers don't give you all the information you wish you had. The only solution for that is something called data sharing, but even a limited paper is typically preferable to an abstract.

In 2015, my colleagues and I examined abstracts from several consecutive cancer national meetings from four to six years back. We wanted to know how many abstracts presented were later published as full papers. This was a laborious project. It involved examining 1,075 abstracts referring to 378 randomized and 697 nonrandomized studies. We found that four to six years after being presented at conference, 25% of randomized trials and 46% of nonrandomized studies had not been published. In other words, anything from one-half to one-fourth of these studies were not published in an arguably reasonable time period.[22] What does this mean? It means that a substantial number of abstracts at a conference end there. All we ever know is the tiny bit of information presented at conferences. It would be like reading a tweet about someone instead of a biography. It isn't quite enough to take the measure of a person.

A final point about conferences worth noting is that the interpretation of results has been shown to change between abstract and published article. Booth and colleagues found this occurred in 10% of all abstract-article pairs, and the most common direction of change was a favorable abstract saying we should adopt a practice changing into an unfavorable conclusion in the paper.[23]

Twenty News Stories, One Patient

Let me end with a final observation. Sometimes when a new therapy is debuted, news outlets feature compelling stories of patients who did really well. Obviously, I wish all patients, including those with the courage to make their story public, the very best. At the same time, I am concerned that the voices we hear in the media do not represent the full results of a therapy, and the stories you don't hear are the ones where patients suffered side effects of therapy. This is unfortunate because the voice of these people is no less important. For this reason, I nodded my head when a senior science and health reporter told me, "Be careful of medical treatments where every news outlet covers the *SAME* patient. If you can only find one person that did well, that might not be such a great therapy."

Conclusion

Focusing only on the one person who did well, spinning a negative study, and hyping a drug tested only in mice are just a few of the ways that our understanding of cancer is distorted. Distortion robs us of free thought. It colors the way we see cancer drug findings and changes how we view the benefits and harms of a therapy. At its worst, it may lead us to make decisions that are not compatible with our true desires. For this reason, understanding its pervasive role in modern media is important.

six

Financial Conflict of Interest

It is difficult to get a man to understand something, when his salary depends
upon his not understanding it.
UPTON SINCLAIR

NOTHING EARNS me fewer friends than my work on financial conflict of interest. In medicine, if you raise the issue of physicians
receiving payments from biopharmaceutical firms, some get annoyed,
irritated, or worse. Yet, because this issue is so important, so intertwined, and so inextricable from the other problems in oncology, I
have been unable to ignore it. It is important to understand this in
order to make sense of what follows in this book. In part III of the
book, I describe clinical trials and their interpretation. Repeatedly, we
will see trials that are flawed—bad comparators, inconclusive endpoints,
or inappropriate design—interpreted favorably. We will see drugs recommended broadly and based on weak or absent evidence (chapter 14),
and physicians cheerleading for marginal products. I believe it is difficult to make sense of these phenomena without understanding the extent of financial ties in the current system. In this chapter, I show you
data that suggest that most of the stakeholders in oncology have financial conflicts with for-profit companies. Personal payments from
drug companies are incredibly common. In chapter 7, I provide data
that suggest these relationships matter. Finally, I outline a solution to
the problem.

Before I delve into data describing the financial ties between physicians and the biopharmaceutical industry, you should understand the

resource that has permitted these studies. In the Affordable Care Act (Obamacare), a clause was added (the Sunshine rule) calling for disclosure, in a federal database, of all money paid from a biopharmaceutical company that sells at least one product in the United States to a doctor authorized to practice medicine. There are some caveats here worth noting. A company has to sell a drug in the United States, so companies with no drugs approved in the United States don't have to disclose. You have to be a doctor who can practice, so PhDs or doctors without a license are not subject to disclosure. In the dataset, there are two types of disclosure—research payments, typically made to a university in order to conduct research, and general payments, which are personal payments made to doctors, usually for consulting or lecturing or advising. Some general payments are for food, drink, and travel. In short, general payments are a direct personal benefit to the doctor, while research payments only provide indirect benefit to the recipient. Throughout this chapter, I discuss general payments only. We can debate the role the biopharmaceutical industry should play in research, but the harms of direct personal payments to physicians are widespread, as I detail in chapter 7.

How Much Money Does the Average Oncologist Receive?

General payments to doctors are ubiquitous. In one of the first studies looking at all medical, surgical, and radiation oncologists—the three major branches of cancer physicians—researchers found, in a single year, 63%, 58%, and 52%, respectively, received money from a pharmaceutical or device company.[1] The size of the payments was generally modest. Medical, surgical, and radiation oncologists had a median payment of $632, $250, and $124, respectively. Remember these numbers. This gives you the lay of the land. This is how conflicted the average doctor in America is. The average doctor, while supremely important to his or her patients, has very minor national influence. Instead, much of cancer medicine   that is, the practice of how cancer is treated—is driven by a smaller cadre of superstars, big fish, thought leaders, or key opinion leaders (KOLs), as they are colloquially known. As we discuss the conflicts present among the big fish, it is instructive to contrast the size of payments against those of the average physician.

What about the Thought Leaders?

Consider just a few of the big fish. Cancer medicine is a complicated field, and each type of cancer has considerable nuance in its management. The FDA approves drugs for cancer, but it does not and cannot provide guidance for the myriad situations encountered in the care of cancer patients. For this reason, tumor-type experts write guidelines specific for each cancer. Guidelines help practicing oncologists in the community make decisions when they realistically cannot keep up with the literature in all topics. Guidelines play another important role: they mandate Medicare, the large federal insurer, to pay for drugs that receive certain recommendations, and insurers often follow in the steps of the Centers for Medicare & Medicaid Services (CMS).[2] For this reason, it is an understatement to say guidelines matter.

In 2016, Aaron Mitchell and colleagues took a close look at the experts who pen perhaps the most influential of these guidelines—those of the National Comprehensive Cancer Network (NCCN).[3] They looked at 125 guideline writers and found that 84% had taken personal payments from pharma, and the average was just over $10,000 ($10,011), with a huge range ($0 to $106,859). Keep in mind—this is for a single year! The doctors who write the NCCN guidelines appear to receive more in payments from pharmaceutical companies than the average cancer doctor in America. Because the weight of these doctors' opinions is greater than the average doctor's, that fact is concerning.

In 2016, my colleagues and I reviewed the financial conflicts of speakers at our national meeting, ASCO (previously discussed in chapter 5).[4] National meetings are important, and the people who speak at the meetings shape the way we think about new products. Our team had a different goal in mind than merely cataloging the conflict (more to come on what we were up to), so we simply recorded the percentage of speakers giving oral presentations who disclosed a conflict of interest. We did this for two consecutive years, 2014 and 2015, but something interesting happened between the meetings. ASCO changed its policy on financial disclosures. The old policy was that speakers disclose conflicts they thought were relevant to their presentation. The new policy was disclosing any financial relationship, irrespective of how the speaker felt about it. In a single year, the percentage of presenters with a financial conflict increased from roughly 50% to 70%. It is highly unlikely the rates of conflict change this quickly. What is more likely is that 20% of speakers had financial ties that they did not think mattered. Since the vast majority of these talks are about the practice of medicine, and since cancer drugs are integral to that practice, it is hard to imagine having a financial tie to a biopharmaceutical maker that would have absolutely no bearing on your presentation.

Oncologists on Social Media

Over the last few years, social media has changed the way we discuss cancer drugs. In blogs, Facebook groups, and on Twitter, doctors, investors, journalists, patient advocates, caregivers, and most importantly, patients are engaged in a dialog about new therapies. In 2016, I got into an argument on Twitter on the subject of whether we (doctors) should speak out about the high prices of cancer drugs and their poor value. There were two factions. One group argued that we have an obligation to speak out. The other group said doctors should stick to medicine, and it wasn't our business to criticize. I thought the second group was taking an absurd, head-in-the-sand position. After an argument that went in circles, I felt compelled to mention the elephant in the room. I looked up the six doctors on the side of "it is a problem," and the five saying "it is not a problem / we should stay out of it" on the open payments database. Then, I tweeted this slide (fig. 6.1):[5]

It was night and day. The doctors who felt it was not a problem had heavy financial ties to the drug industry, and those who did feel it was a problem had nearly no financial ties. Of course, this is just an anecdote, but it got me thinking. This was just one conversation on Twitter.

Financial COI (from Propublica) Among Oncologists on Twitter Who Don't Think Cancer Drug Prices Are Problematic/Not Our Business to Discuss and Those Who Do Think It's a Problem

Not a problem	Yes, a BIG problem
• N = 5	• N = 6
• Median payment = $65,000	• Median payment = $0
	• Range = $0 – $429
• Range = $26,000 – $112,000	

Figure 6.1. Tweet comparing financial conflict of interests among oncologists who argued on Twitter that high drug prices were not a problem or oncologists should not speak out and those who felt it was a problem and oncologists must be vocal.

What if we could look at all of the oncologists on Twitter? What might their conflicts look like? Would it have anything to do with the contents of their tweets?

Led by a then third-year medical student named Derrick Tao, we looked at a systematic set of oncologists based in the United States (where the Sunshine law exists) who were on Twitter. Twitter doesn't provide a list of all oncologists, so we had to build a dataset. After an arduous process where we hand searched tens of thousands of accounts, we ended up with more than 600 hematologist oncologists based in the United States and on Twitter.[6] We found that 72% percent of oncologists on Twitter received personal payments from the pharmaceutical industry. Sixty-six percent received payments in excess of $100, and 44% received in excess of $1,000. The median amount of money received among those with general payments was just over 1,600 dollars.

I found this rate of financial conflicts to be worrying. Doctors on Twitter often comment about new drugs or genetic tests and speak directly to large numbers of patients. This raises the concern that the dialog on twitter may be skewed. Anecdotally, this would explain the rampant hype I see on Twitter but, as the old saying goes, the plural of anecdote is not data.

For this reason, we decided to study Twitter further. We confined ourselves to the most financially conflicted doctors on Twitter—those with at least $1,000 in personal payments. We also focused on the ones who were most active—those with at least 100 tweets. We asked a few questions. First, how often do these doctors tweet about products where they have a financial tie to the maker? How often do they tweet about products where they don't? Are the tweets where a payment has been made more positive and less negative? And, finally, how often do they disclose the conflict to the social media audience?

We found disturbing results:[7] 88% of these doctors tweeted about a drug for which they had a financial tie to the maker, whereas only 2% disclosed those ties. The median payment received was over $13,000 in a single year.

These doctors mentioned specific drugs over 4,000 times in our sampling of their Twitter feeds (we averaged a few hundred tweets per user). Fifty-two percent of the time, they discussed a drug for which they had a financial tie with the manufacturer. You might think that is balanced. Fifty percent of the time they mention a drug with a financial conflict and 50% without a financial conflict. What's the problem? The problem is that 52% reflected the products of, on average, six companies that paid these doctors, and the other half referred to products from any of the other over 350 pharmaceutical companies out there. In other words, 50% of mentions corresponded to just a tiny set of companies in the biopharma universe.

The most concerning finding was about the content of the tweets themselves. My colleagues and I sampled 100 financially conflicted tweets and 100 financially nonconflicted tweets that mentioned a drug and scored them as positive, negative, or neutral. We concealed who the speaker was and whether she or he had a financial conflict. We found that when doctors discussed drugs for which they had received money from the manufacturer, tweets were more likely to be positive (66% vs. 50%; p = 0.02) and less likely to be negative (4% vs. 15%; p = 0.008).

There you have it. Doctors on Twitter are more financially conflicted than the average doctor in America. Many doctors tweet about drugs where a conflict exists, and when they do so, those tweets are more likely to be positive. Disclosure was rare.

In the weeks after our results were published, some readers were curious if I thought pharma was paying these doctors to be on Twitter and say these things. To be honest, I do not think that is happening. My best guess is that the psychological tendencies that predispose one to go on Twitter—like enjoying attention and making short quips— are the same inclinations that predispose someone to take money from pharma. More than money, meeting with pharma reps bathes a doctor with praise and positive reinforcement.

One reader told me something interesting. She said that many celebrities are in a similar situation as doctors—tweeting about a product while being paid by the maker. She said in these situations, some of the celebrities used a hashtag, #sponsored, to convey to readers the potential for bias. I told her this might be among the rare instances when doctors could take a page from the celebrity textbook of ethics.

Patient Advocates

Doctors are not the only group with high rates of financial conflict of interest. Unfortunately, cancer patient advocacy groups often have financial ties to the industry. Why does this matter? A story in *USA Today* made the argument that patient advocacy groups funded by biopharmaceutical companies are notoriously quiet about the rising price of cancer drugs.[8] If you call yourself a patient advocate and are not shouting out about drug prices, then one has to wonder about your loyalties. For interested parties, if you care about the high cost of cancer drugs, check out an advocacy group doing great work: Patients for Affordable Drugs.[9]

In 2016, my colleagues and I examined financial conflicts of interest among cancer patient advocacy groups. We started out by identifying 68 patient advocacy groups endorsed by the National Comprehensive Cancer Network—I keep focusing on the NCCN because it is an influential group, and these were some of the most prominent advocacy groups.

We investigated the disclosed financial links these organizations have to biopharmaceutical companies from their website or from posted financial information, and we found that 75% of groups reported industry sponsorship, 24% did not specify whether they received industry funding or not, and only one organization categorically said it did not take industry funds.[10] What do our results mean? It means the majority of cancer patient organizations have industry ties. One must wonder if they always and only speak on behalf of patients or, as the *USA Today* article suggests, if they fail to comment on important issues like high drug prices as part of a devil's bargain.

Around the Drug Advisory Table

Our discussion of financial conflict in oncology would not be complete without examination of the stakeholders at a single meeting: the Oncology Drug Advisory Committee (ODAC) meeting at the FDA.

To understand the ODAC, you need to know that the FDA can approve and reject drugs all by itself and often does this. Occasionally, for drugs with a very uncertain risk-benefit balance, the FDA is empowered to convene a panel of national experts to advise it. The advice is nonbinding and the FDA doesn't have to take it, but the meetings are open to the public, and they permit the FDA and experts to put their reasoning out there for all to view.

Although the ODAC is nonbinding, the FDA often follows its advice. In fact, stock prices rise and fall on an ODAC vote, which suggests that the decision matters. For this reason, one would want all of the participants in that meeting to be devoid of any alternative motives or biases. Just as in a court of law, where the defendant cannot pay the judge, so too the corporate sponsor of the drug should probably not fund any of the ODAC participants.

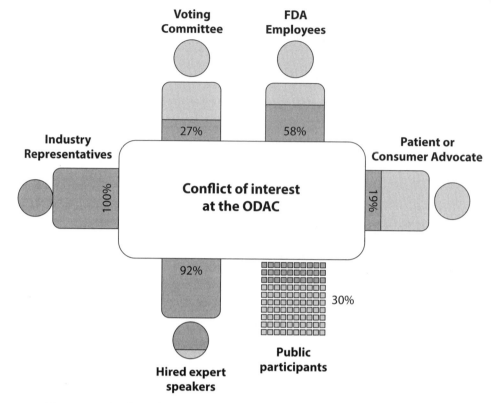

Figure 6.2. Conflict of interest among the voting members of the Oncology Drug Advisory Committee (ODAC)

In figure 6.2, I have depicted the six groups that participate in the ODAC. They are employees of the FDA, the voting members of ODAC, a patient or consumer advocate, representatives from the industry, a hired expert speaker, and public participants. Let's take each one in turn, and examine whether they have any past, present, or future conflicts with the pharmaceutical industry.

Employees of the US FDA give one of the key presentations of the meeting and ultimately decide if the controversial drug is approved. By law, employees of the Food and Drug Administration cannot receive payments from pharmaceutical companies concurrent with their duties, and for good reason.

Enter Jeff Bien. Jeff was an OHSU resident who came to me looking for a project. Knowing what I know about the FDA, I asked Jeff to assemble a list of medical reviewers at the FDA from a few years back and then look up where they work now. My question was, even though FDA employees aren't conflicted *at the time of their employment,* is there a revolving door between FDA and pharma?

Building the list of names was difficult. They were all in the public record, available on the FDA website, but navigating the website is not intuitive, and Jeff had to work hard. We joked that getting this information was like eating a pomegranate. Yes, there is fruit in there, but you have to work for it.

Jeff's results were concerning.[11] He found 55 reviewers who served as medical reviewers between 2001 and 2010. When he searched for these people in 2016, he found 26 had left the FDA. Of these 26, Jeff could link 15 (58%) to a subsequent job either working for or consulting for pharma. This percentage was high and suggested that the most common position after being a reviewer at the FDA is pharma. The revolving door spins.

Employees from the FDA didn't like our findings. They did their own analysis and found 10/27 employees (37%) went to work for or consult for pharma. Here, I have to add a bit of explanation. The FDA certainly has a better ability to sort out the denominator, as the agency has access to the old records, but the numerator was created by Google searching. Nothing fancy, the same way you would try to track down a high school friend. The FDA might be right that we are off by one in the denominator, but I suspect Jeff is better at Google searching than the agency is, and that is why the FDA is wrong about the 10. It is 15, and the rate is closer to 58%.[12] In fact, during the writing of this book, Charles Piller, an investigative journalist, replicated this analysis and found 68% (11/16) reviewers who leave the FDA work for or consult for pharma.[13] However, the overall point remains the same. Whether it is 37% or 58% or 68%, that is still a big revolving door. The concern remains.

What is the concern? It isn't that these reviewers are engaged in some sort of quid pro quo. Nothing that nefarious. The concern is that if you knew you had a 40% to 70% chance of working for the person on the other side of the table, would you really want to regulate hard? Do you really want to be thought of as difficult? Or do you want to try to push drugs through? Do you want to be thought of as agreeable? If I knew there was a 58% chance I would end up working at the University of Pittsburgh, for example, it is a safe bet that I wouldn't be too tough on that university.

The issue of the revolving door between government and industry is not limited to health care. Other examples include the Securities and Exchange Commission and Goldman Sachs, the Environmental Protection Agency and chemical companies, and the list goes on.

Now let's turn to the voting members of the ODAC. In 2006, Peter Lurie and colleagues published a review in *JAMA* that looked at ODAC meetings from 2001 to 2004 and showed that more than 70% had at least one voting member with a financial conflict.[14] In the wake of this paper, the FDA sought reform. Rates of *active* financial conflict among voting members declined over time and were absent in 2014 (0/20).[15] At the same time, these voting members still had *prior* conflicts to the companies. A recent analysis found that 27% of voting members previously received money from the sponsor company.[16] The authors of that paper assure us that this did not change the vote, and I actually believe them. It would be like saying this dash of salt did not make the chicken taste any different, after you had soaked the chicken overnight in a soy sauce marinade. In other words, conflict is so common and pervasive, I doubt this one extra bit makes a difference. At the same time, I suspect the chicken would taste different if you didn't use any soy sauce at all.

The next group to talk about is the industry. The pharmaceutical company makes the case that its product should be approved, and—no surprise—has always supported approval. The company is allowed to invite an expert to speak on behalf of its product. Companies often select a giant in oncology. Someone with sterling credentials, huge curricula vitae, and expertise beyond question, but what about his or her conflicts?

Now remember, because the Affordable Care Act's Sunshine clause does not apply to companies that do not have a product on the market, we cannot know exactly how many experts were paid to defend those products. Yet, my colleagues and I found that 92% of experts invited by the industry had received a payment from a biopharmaceutical company (though as I note, we could not identify the full number who received money from that company). Nevertheless, let me restate the finding: 92% had received money from some company. The median payment was $35,000.[17] I began this chapter with talk about big fish. Here they are. The major voices in oncology are heavily paid by the industry. We performed an additional analysis, asking if the amount of money these experts receive correlated with their publication and citation record (that is, the measure of success in academic medicine). We found a strong correlation, which begs the question: which came first? (More to come on this.)

Now, let us turn to the last two ODAC groups. First is the patient/consumer advocate. The patient advocate is presumably there to speak on behalf of what patients want. In an analysis of drug advisory meetings from 2009 to 2012, 19% of meetings had an advocate with a financial conflict of interest.[18]

The sixth and final group of ODAC is the public. The public is allowed an opportunity for an open microphone. My colleagues and I examined the conflict among 103 members of the audience who spoke at these meetings. Audience members may not be doctors, so we had to rely on self-disclosed conflicts at the start of their remarks. We found 31 speakers (30.1%) reported financial associations, such as travel funding or funding from any organization they were affiliated with. Moreover, more than 92% of speakers argued the drug should be approved; only 6% said it shouldn't, and 2% were neutral.[19] By the way, of those who spoke against approving the drug, none had a financial conflict.

What does this mean? If you look around the table at the drug advisory meeting, all parties have high past, present, or future rates of financial ties to the drug industry. It is challenging to think of the forum as an impartial hearing of the risks and potential benefits of products when many of the participants derive substantial income, at some point during their career, from the pharmaceutical companies. In short, the worry is that the meeting is elaborate theater incapable of being truly critical of cancer drugs that deliver poor gains with tremendous toxicity.

Conclusion

Putting this all together and looking at figure 6.2 again, you see that financial conflict is the marinade, and decisions surrounding the approval, use, and payment of cancer drugs are the chicken. The entire cancer ecosystem is soaking in the industry's influence, and it is hard to believe this does not curry favor. Yet, the information I have portrayed in this chapter is merely to show you the lay of the land. In the next chapter, I address the key questions: Why are these financial ties problematic? And, what can be done to address the problem?

SEVEN

The Harms of Financial Conflicts and How to Rehabilitate Medicine

For where your treasure is, there will your heart be also.
MATTHEW 6:21

IN THE first part of our discussion of financial conflict, I let the data speak for itself. We analyzed studies from medical journals and found that financial ties are widespread among all stakeholders in the broad cancer arena. Financial ties are present among doctors, patient advocates, certain vocal patient advocates, and in the subsequent lives of regulators of the FDA. Here I am going to provide evidence for why these conflicts matter and what we can do about them. Before I do that, I want to give you some perspective.

Financial Conflicts within and outside of Medicine

Let me begin by reminding you of one group with significant financial conflicts—the experts in cancer medicine. The experts are the ones who speak at national meetings, write the guidelines (which mandate Medicare to pay), write editorials, and lend their expert perspectives at FDA meetings. In chapter 6, I provided data that show the majority of these doctors are conflicted. Their incentives are not small. In many cases, they rival the annual household income in America.

In biomedicine, especially for diseases with a limited amount of very knowledgeable people on the topic (for example, cancer), the power of an expert is tremendous. Experts are judge, jury, and executioner when it comes to how cancer should be treated. Moreover, the evidence for many cancers has limited randomized trial data and far more historically controlled or uncontrolled trials and observational data (see chapter 9). These forms of data are more uncertain. Therefore, experts are making powerful proclamations in a gray zone.

In every walk of life, we understand that human beings, no matter how honest or pure, are driven by incentives. In cases where people act as judge or jury, we prefer them to be without conflict. For instance, you would not be happy if the judge in a court of law was paid by the defense. You wouldn't want your senators or president receiving payments from Blue Cross Blue Shield while they simultaneously worked on health insurance policy. Similarly, you would think doctors in these privileged roles should also be without conflict.

In an article I wrote with Kevin De Jesus appearing in the *Hastings Center Report,* a bioethics journal, we argue that political corruption and medical financial conflict were similar but treated completely differently.[1]

Consider the cases of former Virginia governor, Bob McDonnell, and the former New York State assemblyman, Sheldon Silver. Both were politicians who were convicted based on the honest services fraud statute. Because of a Supreme Court ruling limiting the scope of that charge, both have been set free. Yet, in my nonexpert opinion, what they did remains troubling, and it is possible that future jurisprudence will see things differently.

McDonnell accepted over $100,000 in gifts, and he just happened to extend favors to the gift giver, including use of the governor's mansion.[2] He was charged with misuse of his position in exchange for those gifts. Silver was the New York State speaker of the house since 1994. He also worked for a personal injury law firm, a job for which he received a large personal income. One of the ways the law firm made considerable money was from prosecuting cases where asbestos may have caused mesothelioma. Asbestos exposure, once common in the United States, is linked to this rare tumor. People with mesothelioma were referred to the firm from a mesothelioma specialist at Columbia University named Dr. Robert Taub. Nothing so far seems off. A doctor

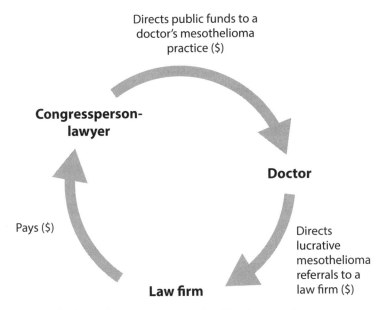

Directs public funds to a doctor's mesothelioma practice ($)

Congressperson-lawyer

Doctor

Pays ($)

Directs lucrative mesothelioma referrals to a law firm ($)

Law firm

Figure 7.1. The flow of money in a case of political corruption

who sees mesothelioma patients may direct many of his patients to a personal injury law firm. The problem is that the doctor in question just happened to be the recipient of research funding that Sheldon Silver, in his capacity as speaker of the house, administered.[3] Using the case of Silver, we diagrammed the relationship (fig. 7.1).

Putting aside the legal nuances, the fact that both of these men were prosecuted and convicted is indicative that many Americans don't feel comfortable with this relationship. These politicians have a fiduciary duty to act in the public interest. That means the welfare of the public should guide their decision making for work-related actions while in office. In both cases, there were some work-related actions made (for example, use of the governor's mansion and dispensing funds for meso-thelioma research) that created a closed financial loop focused on ben-efiting the political leaders and private industry without a clear benefit to the public they served. In both cases, we are genuinely unsure if this was a quid pro quo or just a coincidence. A juror in the case of Mr. Silver summed it up nicely. She thought the money directed to the me-sothelioma doctor may just be "goodwill."[1]

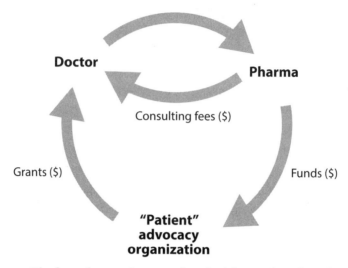

Heavily prescribes a costly drug when data
about it is unclear; advocates for the drug to be
recommended in medical guidelines ($)

Doctor

Pharma

Consulting fees ($)

Grants ($)

Funds ($)

**"Patient"
advocacy
organization**

Figure 7.2. The flow of money in cases of medical financial conflict of interest

In fact, the politicians could argue that they just happened to favor these people and happened to receive gifts or money, but that the two were unrelated. Yet, despite this, I think many of us would prefer that persons with fiduciary responsibility not put themselves in such questionable arrangements.

Now, contrast this with doctors in medicine. Doctors have a fiduciary duty to act always and inexorably in a patient's best interest. In fact, they take such an oath. Yet, they routinely put themselves in closed financial loop situations (fig. 7.2). Just as in the case of the politicians, doctors can easily say, "These activities don't affect each other; just because I receive payments from pharmaceutical companies does not mean I use their drug more." Just because the patient advocacy organization accepts money from pharma does not make it unwilling to speak out on cancer drug costs.

The difference between politicians and doctors is that politicians have not been extensively studied, whereas doctors have. If anything, the data on doctors is stronger, but you don't hear too many calls for financial conflicts to be policed the same way. Why do we treat these situations differently? Perhaps part of the answer to that question has to do with the fact that the public is distrustful of politicians, while doctors have always benefited from positive public perception.

Proof That Conflicts Matter

Recent studies suggest that pharmaceutical company payments to doctors deliver value to pharma. But before seeing that data, just ask yourself: would a multi-billion-dollar organization really spend billions of dollars on something if it didn't improve its bottom line? It would be both illogical and bad business if companies paid doctors sizable sums and did not benefit.

In 2016, Fleischman and colleagues showed that, for oral anticoagulant drugs and non-insulin diabetic drugs, the two most prescribed (and marketed) classes of drugs, greater payments from the pharmaceutical industry to physicians were associated with greater prescribing of marketed versus generic alternatives at a regional level.[4] Every $13 paid to doctors was associated with around three months of extra use of a marketed drug. Of course, given the price of some of these medicines and the profit margins on them, that is likely a good return on investment.

That same year, Yeh and colleagues found this held true at the individual doctor level. They looked at the percent of instances a doctor prescribed a brand name over a cheaper (and probably equally effective) statin. For every $10,000 in payments, doctors seemed to increase prescribing brand name statins by 1%.[5]*

Conflict of interest isn't just about receiving money. DeJong and colleagues looked at whether having even a single meal paid for by pharmaceutical companies would influence prescribing practices. They found that doctors who got a single meal were more likely to prescribe an expensive statin over cheaper ones (odds ratio [OR], 1.18; 95% confidence interval [CI], 1.17–1.18), an expensive beta blocker over cheaper

---

* During the writing of this book, Aaron Mitchell and colleagues published several articles extending these findings and establishing that payments go hand in hand with prescribing patterns for costly cancer drugs.

ones (OR, 1.70; 95% CI, 1.69–1.72), an expensive blood pressure pill over cheaper ones (OR, 1.52; 95% CI, 1.51–1.53), and a pricey antidepressant over cheaper ones (OR, 2.18; 95% CI, 2.13–2.23).[6]

Conflict of interest doesn't only affect the average doctor; it also affects the experts and key opinion leaders. In 2007, a meta-analysis suggested that a popular diabetes drug, rosiglitazone (Avandia), might increase heart attacks. Wang and colleagues explored articles commenting on that topic. They found that authors who had received payments from diabetes drug makers were more likely to think the link was overblown and more likely to recommend use of the drug.[7] This was true even for the authors of opinion articles—those that shape the interpretation of medical data.

Fugh-Berman and colleagues found that after a randomized trial contradicted the widespread use of hormone replacement therapy (for a full discussion, see my first book, *Ending Medical Reversal*), some articles attacked the applicability of the randomized trial, arguing that it didn't apply to individuals. They claimed that observational studies were superior to randomized trials for guiding clinical decisions (a highly debatable proposition). Could you guess that these opinions went hand in hand with financial conflicts of interest?[8]

Some argue that these aforementioned studies do not prove that payments caused the behavior. Strictly speaking, they are correct. At the same time, when it comes to political corruption, we don't have studies that *prove* causality, yet many observers recognize it as problematic. Here, in contrast with governmental corruption, we have an empirically proven link. If anything, our concern and attitude should be stronger.

What Do We Do about Conflict in Medicine?

Meanwhile, what do we do about conflict? In reality, we do very little. Mostly, we ask doctors to disclose their conflicts. Thanks to the Affordable Care Act, we can study the problem, but most patients don't look up whether their doctors have conflict of interest. In a rare and highly publicized incident during the writing of this book, José Baselga, the prominent physician mentioned in chapter 5, resigned from his position after reports were made of large, undisclosed conflicts alongside extremely positive rhetoric about a company's products.[9,10] Yet, ousting remains unusual. Later during the publication of the book, Dr. Baselga was hired in a coveted leadership position by AstraZeneca. The penalty for undisclosed conflict does not seem too onerous. In a paper published in *JAMA Oncology*, my colleagues and I demonstrated that much of our disclosure policies amounted to no more than a token gesture.[11]

In chapter 6, I explained the percentage of speakers at the national meeting who disclosed ties to pharmaceutical companies in 2014 and 2015. Now I can tell you what we were really after. In that same paper, we also examined how these conflicts were disclosed. We watched videos of the presenters and used a stopwatch to time how long the authors left up their disclosure slides (where they report any financial ties). We also counted the number of words on each slide.

Now, in order to appreciate our findings, you need to know that the average person reads about 3.8 words per second. A proofreader, who is engaging with the text, can do about 3.3 words per second. Feeling generous, we said a conference attendee could read four words per second. With that cutoff, we found that 38% of the slides were flashed faster than a human being could read. Figure 7.3 shows a graph of the words per second for each presenter (each bar represents one presenter). Some slides were flashed as fast as 15 to 20 words per second. It seems that when it comes to disclosing conflicts of interest (COIs), our conference efforts are a token disclosure—an empty act meant to say we are doing something when nothing is being done.

Does Conflict Hurt the Authors?

Recently I heard someone remark that doctors who receive industry funds are penalized academically. Because there is a stigma against the pharmaceutical industry, careers are hurt, the argument went. It struck me as an odd claim, but interesting, provocative, and testable.

My colleagues and I wanted to know if personal ties to the industry

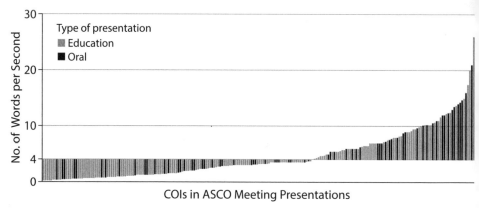

Figure 7.3. Conflicts of Interest (COIs) for oral presentations at the 2015 Annual Meeting of the American Society of Clinical Oncology (ASCO). Reading ability was four words per second or below in 62% of presentations and above four words per second in 38% of presentations. Used with permission by *JAMA Oncology.*

were helpful for one's career or a hindrance. We built a dataset of more than 400 physicians who published in top journals, and extracted their financial conflicts of interest. We performed an analysis to see the relationship between personal payments and publications. We found that for every $10,000 received, a physician published 1.99 more papers.[12] Adjusting for seniority, prior publications, and research funds from the industry, the association persisted (0.84 papers per $10,000). What does this mean? It appears that receiving personal payments from companies is a boost to one's career, not a hindrance.

The *New England Journal of Medicine* (NEJM)

The *NEJM* is the highest-impact-factor general medical journal (that is, the most heavily cited) and was the finest medical journal for a long time. In my mind, editorial policies over the last decade on topics such as conflict of interest, data sharing, independent audit, and transparency have all led to its decline,[13] though it remains influential.

The changing politics of the *NEJM* serve as a bellwether for conflict of interest. During the 1980s and 1990s, *NEJM* editors Arnold Relman and Jerome Kassirer were concerned about the pervasive role of the pharmaceutical industry and conflict of interest. Relman wrote a prescient article warning of a medical-industrial complex,[14] which threatened the knowledge and practice of medicine. Kassirer was also concerned. In his memoir, *Unanticipated Outcomes,* he writes:

> What has become clear is that some drug and device companies have deliberately biased clinical trials by hiding inconvenient and unfavorable results, failed to conceal randomization in blinded studies, excluded subjects selectively after randomization, and used inexperienced physicians to enroll test subjects and carry out studies. In endeavoring to publish data favorable to editorial and regulatory approval they refused to give all study data even to the principal investigator of studies, required that investigators sign gag clauses promising never to release data, and zealously guarded the option of finalizing manuscripts destined for journal submission. Even when required to provide data when their published conclusions were openly criticized, some stonewalled, produced heavily redacted data sheets, and agreed to perform follow-up studies but then never did. All of these tactics are well documented, and nearly all major pharmaceutical and device companies were guilty of some of these flawed practices. The consequences of these subterfuges were serious; dangerous drugs were approved or left on the market too long; many drugs initially considered to have important therapeutic properties were later found to produce no benefit and thus subjected patients only to adverse events. Meanwhile the companies made millions in sales; and the public was paying for useless and dangerous drugs.[15]

Relman and Kassirer understood the influence of the pharmaceutical industry on reliable scientific information. Of course, it is almost self-evident that allowing the design, conduct, and reporting of data to be run by the same entity that stands to make or lose a billion dollars is ripe for bias. Recognition of this problem, however, largely ended at the *NEJM* with the tenure of Jeffrey Drazen.

As editor-in-chief of the *NEJM*, Drazen changed regulations to allow authors of reviews and editorials to hold monetary conflicts.

Now, restrictions are limited to $10,000 in conflict (a tidy sum). Moreover, during Drazen's term, the journal published a three-part series on financial conflict of interest, which essentially argued that the concern regarding financial conflict was overblown. In response, Robert Steinbrook, former *NEJM* national correspondent, Jerome Kassirer, and Marcia Angell, another former *NEJM* editor-in-chief, wrote a blistering reply, entitled, "Justifying Conflicts of Interest in Medical Journals: A Very Bad Idea."[16]

In 2017, a colleague and I studied conflict of interest among editorialists at top journals. We picked these articles because of the high potential for bias to play a role. We chose the three highest-impact factor journals and audited them. We found that 18% of articles had a financial conflict with the drug or device discussed. Notably, we found three articles that appear to be in violation of *NEJM's* rule, with payments in excess of $10,000 for the drug or device discussed.[17] Our results suggest that roughly one in five editorials at the very top of biomedicine have an author with a conflict.

Relaxing rules around financial conflicts for editorialists is deeply problematic. A favorable editorial can go a long way to promote a practice or intervention, whereas a damning one seeds widespread doubt. Since editorials are essentially the author's opinion regarding research, the ability to come to a favorable or disparaging conclusion are often both possible. For this reason, impartiality is not just desired, it is necessary, and the shifting attitudes at the *NEJM* are emblematic of the trends that have shaped biomedicine over the last 40 years.

The Solution

All of this is a prelude to the solution. If one were not aware of the information presented in chapter 6 and 7, the solution to the problem would sound draconian or even punitive. However, the solution is designed to shift the compass of cancer care discussion back to the patient. The solution is that doctors should not be able to receive personal payments from for-profit companies that sell health care products. This means no pharma meals, no device maker honoraria, no consulting fees from test makers. Disclosure is not the solution; divestiture is—severing the ties.

It isn't hard. FDA employees have to do it—at least while they work for the agency. Judges have to do it. It is possible for oncology and medicine, in general, to embrace this solution.

One of the persistent objections I hear is that banning payments from pharma would end collaboration and innovation. That argument is flawed. First, I am not proposing a ban on research payments from the industry that go to universities and fund clinical research. This can continue, but the personal payments to doctors have no good purpose. I am also not proposing a ban on speaking with or interacting with pharma. I've spoken at pharmaceutical companies and not received reimbursement or compensation. I have also coauthored papers with dozens of students, residents, and fellows over the years, and in no case did any of my collaborators pay me $10,000 for an hour of my time (not even sure I got a cup of coffee). In fact, just like working with students is a part of my job, working on trials is part of the job of a trialist. Clearly, working together and paying each other are not equivalent.

I'll also note that the rules against conflict are stricter when you work for a pharma company than if you work for Memorial Sloan Kettering Cancer Center. If you work for Pfizer, for example, the company will not be happy if you consult for Merck. That imbalance makes no sense.

There are other complementary solutions:

1. Professional organizations like ASCO and ASH (American Society of Hematology) should end financial relationships with pharmaceutical companies. They should raise revenue through dues, like most organizations, and learn to tighten the belt. Not every meeting has to be the pinnacle of opulence.
2. Patient advocacy organizations should not accept money from pharmaceutical companies. If they do, they should call themselves pharmaceutical advocacy organizations (and at times, their behavior is consistent with that). These organizations often call for the approval of unproven or marginal drugs, criticize

programs that push for lower costs or cost-effective care, and are strangely silent on the issue of high drug prices.

3. We have to rethink one of the fundamental misaligned incentives that I did not cover in-depth, which is that cancer doctors are paid a percentage of the IV medication they administer (those Medicare Part B drugs from chapter 4). This creates a perverse incentive to use costlier drugs. It must be eliminated.

4. The people who write the guidelines should be without conflicts of interest.

5. We need some rules governing when and where former FDA officials can work for or consult for the pharmaceutical industry. I don't know whether a lifetime ban is needed or if a cooling-off period of a few years would do. Obviously, this will disincentivize working for the FDA, which is already an underappreciated job. A compensatory measure would be to pay reviewers fairly, on par with what they would earn in the private sector.

6. The party that designs, conducts, collects, analyzes, reports, and presents data on cancer drugs should not be the party that stands to make billions of dollars if the trial is positive. The current system of industry-sponsored research—where a for-profit company designs, conducts, analyzes, writes, and reports results—is grievously flawed. More to come on this topic in chapter 14.

These six rules would push us a long way toward a more logical, honest, and aligned cancer system. That said, I understand that moving from the current world, where conflict is ubiquitous, to this proposed world is a huge jump. Good policy is incremental. For that reason, Vincent Rajkumar and I proposed a set of solutions that could happen tomorrow.[18] Let me highlight two.

One, we argue that the use of medical writers should be abandoned. Medical writers are people who provide service-for-hire help with manuscript preparation. These people are good at their job, and, unfortunately, this is a bad thing. Some medical writers may be skilled in playing up the benefits of a drug and minimizing the harms. Moreover, if you put your name on a manuscript and said you wrote it, you probably should have. This is the standard we hold college students too, why not physicians?

Two, we argue that professional organizations like ASCO and ASH should fully disclose their funding sources. Transparency has many purposes, as discussed before, and most importantly, it is a prerequisite to study the problem of conflict of interest. When it comes to professional organizations, they remain a black box.

These Aren't Bad People

I think I should state clearly that I do not believe the problem with conflict of interest, even regarding the oversized and distorting role of the biopharmaceutical industry, is a result of bad people. For the most part, people in these roles are just as decent and honest as anyone else. They probably see the good in what they do. They may be oblivious to many of these facts.

The real problems are the incentives. The policies that are implemented at these institutions push people to act the way they do. They foster and encourage financial conflict among doctors, who then come to see the silver lining in marginal drugs, and may even ignore the harms, costs, and toxicities. The role of the financial incentives is not like a light switch that acts in an all or nothing manner. Rather, it acts more like a dimmer switch, darkening the room. This results in biomedicine doing less for the best interest of patients and more for the best interest of profits.

Conclusion

We are now in a period of history where physicians who interpret the data for medical products also happen to prescribe these same medical products to patients. They are being paid by both the patient and by the manufacturers of these products. This creates a tension, simply because the best interests of the manufacturers and patients occasionally, perhaps even often, diverge. There are no well-established rules of evidence-based medicine to guide these doctors (though in future chapters I will offer some candidate rules), and most decision making occurs in the gray. As in all human endeavors, when someone has to make decisions in the face of uncertainty, and you want them to make decisions that are just, honest, and virtuous, you have to pay them in a manner that doesn't push them one way or the other. This is why judges get salaries and are not paid by the defense. This is also why pharmaceutical companies do not allow their employees to be paid by other pharmaceutical companies. Yet, this does not occur in medicine, particularly among its leaders. The solution to the current problem is to fix the broken incentive structure. There is no reason why the costs of health care, which is nearly 20% of US GDP, should be meted out under conditions that even a first-year psychology student would see as a recipe for disaster.

[EIGHT]
Will Precision Oncology Save Us?

I prefer physicians . . . [who] do not highly praise their own remedies, for they well know that the work must praise the master, not the master praise his work. They well know that words and chatter do not help the sick nor cure them.

PARACELSUS

IN THE introduction, we saw how one school of thought, one fad— the idea that curing cancer only required a higher dose of chemo-therapy—dominated cancer medicine and led to widespread use of an ineffective therapy. In the modern world, we have also become seduced by a singular idea that cancer will soon be brought to its knees thanks to advances in whole genome sequencing. Indeed, we increasingly hear the message that, while cancer care has been thus far suboptimal, we are on the verge of a personalized breakthrough. In this chapter, I discuss personalized, or precision, cancer medicine. What does the term *personalized cancer care* really mean? What are its prospects? And how can we test it?

Is It Personalized or Precision Oncology?

I prefer the term *precision oncology* to describe the new movement in cancer therapy for the same reason that former National Institutes of Health (NIH) director and Nobel laureate Harold Varmus prefers it. Varmus argued that the doctor who took care of his father, in an era before genomics and other technological advances, personalized the care to his dad.[1] Varmus is correct. Physicians have always tailored the care for an individual person, drawing from general principles, experience, basic science, and data from populations. Doctors have always performed personalized medicine. What's new is the widespread use of genomics to inform therapeutic decisions. For this reason, going forward, I will only use the term *precision oncology.*

What Is Precision Oncology?

In my mind, and I am going to support this with data, precision oncology means prescribing drugs to cancer patients based on the results of genetic sequencing, RNA sequencing, RNA measurement, protein measurement, or other -*omics* testing. If that sounds like gobbledygook, it basically means that doctors will come up with specific drugs or combinations for each patient using the new tools of genomics and molecular biology.

Now, here are the data. Robert Peter Gale, a senior oncologist, and I sampled the biomedical literature for use of the term *precision oncology* at three different time points: 2005–2010, 2013, and 2016.* We coded all articles in terms of how the authors used the phrase. We found a few things.[2]

First, in the modern era (2016), 80% of the studies referred to precision oncology as the use of -*omics* (like genomics) testing to prescribe therapy. In other words, regardless of where the cancer began, be it breast, prostate, or pancreatic, we should be able to sequence the genome and decide on a treatment. That definition fits with how I conceptualize precision oncology, and I will use that going forward.

We also noticed that the definition has changed. In the earliest period, *precision oncology* mostly referred to therapy that targeted some malfunctioning cancer protein (for example, a pill like imatinib; see chapter 1) that was applied to all people with a given disease. In the 2013 period, *precision oncology* referred to a molecular test used in a single cancer type (such as lung cancer or colon cancer patients) to decide which patients should get a certain drug. For instance, if you had

---

* Since the phrase was more commonly used over time, we had to use a range of years for the first data point so that all three time slices had a roughly equal sample size.

lung cancer and an activating mutation in EGFR (epidermal growth factor receptor), you should get erlotinib. By 2016, *precision oncology* shifted to the use of next generation sequencing or other *-omics* to treat cancer irrespective of the tissue of origin. *Precision oncology* is an imprecise term over time, it seems.

Definitions are important. They frame our discussions. We have to keep them consistent over time, so that we can accurately judge whether promises materialize.

Is Precision Oncology Common?

Using the 2016 definition, precision oncology is vastly popular. Major academic medical centers have sequenced tens of thousands of patients. One group, called GENIE, has sequenced 18,000 patients.[3] Private companies are in on the action. Biotech companies such as Foundation Medicine and Guardiant have sequenced thousands of cancer patients' tumors (90,000 and 20,000 tumors, respectively).[4,5] Since Foundation Medicine is priced at $5,800 per patient, its revenue might be as high as $500 million.[6]

What Will It Take for Precision Oncology to Work?

Precision oncology holds the idea that we will sequence cancer patients' genomes, and irrespective of the origin of that cancer (breast or colon or lung), we will find mutations against which targeted drugs can be given. For instance, people with several different cancer types may all share a mutation in a gene called *B-Raf* (*B-Raf* proto-oncogene, serine/threonine kinase) that is able to be treated with vemurafenib or dabrafenib (two inhibitors of *B-Raf*).

For precision oncology to work, sequencing has to (1) lead to matches between patient tumors and drugs (ideally, a considerable number of matches); (2) lead to tumor shrinkage in matched patients (ideally, total tumor shrinkage); and (3) lead to longer survival in patients compared to patients who had not undergone sequencing but instead had a doctor prescribe drugs the old-fashioned way (which does lead to some responses). Unfortunately, it turns out the data for these points are uncertain or unfavorable.

How Many Patients Match to Treatment?

I have to admit this is a moving target. The easiest way to match a lot of patients is to be very loose about what defines a match. Moreover, as more drugs develop, there will be more matches. Still, a look at the best-published estimates of match rate (as of the summer of 2017) is sobering.

One large ongoing federal study of precision oncology, called the NCI Match trial, reports that, as of March 12, 2017, only 495/4702 (10.5%) of patients who underwent Next Generation Sequencing (NGS) were paired with therapy.[7] That means that 89.5% did not match. For those who do not match, these kinds of treatment strategies cannot help. A 10% match rate is poor, and if it is not improved upon, the entire idea may falter.

Of course, the NCI Match is only the most well-known effort. Individual cancer centers have their own matching programs. One center reported that as many as 25% of its patients matched.[8] The issue with this is that the center used a loose definition of *match*. It gave a drug to a patient if there was some laboratory evidence it would hit the mutation and not necessarily if the drug was approved for that mutation or meant primarily for that mutation. Moreover, the NCI Match had a predefined set of matches that would be accepted, but this study did not have the same rigor in its design. A predefined set of matches is needed to ensure that investigators do not get desperate and keep searching for matches, especially poor-quality ones.

If You Match, Does Your Tumor Shrink?

If you match to a molecular therapy, do you experience tumor shrinkage? The recent publication of a trial called MOSCATO-1 (yes, that does sound delicious) looks to answer this question. Just over 1,000 patients were enrolled with the intention of undergoing sequencing.

Almost 200 (n = 199), or roughly 20%, were paired with a drug, and 22 patients achieved a partial or complete response.

In short, there was a roughly 2% chance (22/1000) that if you enrolled in this study, you would experience tumor shrinkage because of a matched therapy. The reader may not know this, but that is low. As a general rule, a 10%–20% response rate is the response rate for an old-fashioned cytotoxic therapy in people with relapsed cancers.

If You Send Your Cancer for Two Different Tests, Do You Get Paired with the Same Drug?

All this time, we have taken something for granted. We are assuming there is some reliability to the results of genetic sequencing (sequenced results that somehow tell us something fundamental about the patient's cancer). One simple way to test this is to send the same patient's samples in (either blood or tissue) for multiple tests.

As of the writing of this book, I am aware of three studies that did this.[9-11] If you combine the studies, the results are troubling. Only 20% (36/217) of the mutations found in samples from 56 patients were found by both tests. By combining the results of the three studies, we can find the answer to another question: how often did these two different tests suggest the same drug? That happened 25% of the time (9/36).[9]

Some of this disagreement may be because mutations in the blood are different from those in the tumor. However, even when two tests of tumor tissue are compared, there are marked differences.[12]

What about the Wonderful Anecdotes?

These facts conflict with the persistent anecdotes that fill newspapers, magazines, and the nightly news. Unfortunately, all these stories merely consider the tip of the iceberg—the success stories.

What happens if you look systematically at all anecdotes? In 2015, Dr. Andrae Vandross and I looked at the entire oncology literature and could find 32 examples of precision oncology success stories, or super responders. We found that many of these cases seemed odd. A patient did very well with a paired drug—that was true—but this person had already done exceptionally well prior to the "precise" therapy. If a person far outlived the average life expectancy before he or she got sequenced, one wonders how much the new drug did, and how much the prolonged survival is due to the fact that the individual has a naturally slow-growing or sensitive tumor.[13]

We also found that many of these reports omitted crucial data. Twenty percent did not report how many treatments the patient had received previously. Sixteen percent did not say whether the tumors shrank or not (that is, if there was a response). Sixty-two percent did not report the number of patients treated similarly (how many patients were sequenced) before the super response occurred. This is vitally important, as it tells you how many people bore the expenses and false promises to find one super responder.

In 2017, Jia Luo, Go Nishikawa, and I updated this analysis. This time we found 180 cases.[14] We made a number of similar observations and pushed our findings further. We found that only a third of patients highlighted in these success stories had a complete response, and to me this is what you need to really be a super responder. The median duration of response was 14 months, which is not bad, but the median duration of response to a prior line of therapy, when reported, was 8 months. Eight months is a fairly high number, suggesting that many of the patients' tumors have indolent biology.

One type of analysis that can help in these situations is the *Von Hoff ratio* of progression-free survival (PFS). The Von Hoff ratio states that one might feel more confident of a drug's benefit if the PFS on the drug was 1.3 times as long as the PFS on the prior treatment. Applying this criterion to all the cases, we found just under 50% met the criterion. Keep in mind, this isn't a very stringent criterion, and less than half meet the mark. In my mind, it means that many of these cases are not as good as the ones that make the news.

We also looked at financial conflicts of interest. We found that authors with a financial tie to the drug or genetic test used were more likely to omit information than those without such ties. Of course, it is easy to declare success and go unchallenged the less information you provide.

There is one final thing you should think about. It is called the *Fermi estimate*. Enrico Fermi was a renowned mathematician who came up with a clever way to estimate challenging problems. It is often used in interviews for consulting jobs. The basic method is to estimate a complex quantity by breaking it into smaller parts and rounding all those parts to the nearest order of magnitude. An order of magnitude is the nearest 10th, 100th, 1,000th, and so on depending on the number. For example, the nearest order of magnitude to 88 is 100. What the method does is allow a lot of random error of estimation (too high or too low) to cancel out.

If you applied this to super responders you would get the following: 100,000 people have been sequenced (nearest order of magnitude), and we could find 100 (nearest order of magnitude) published cases. This would suggest that fewer than 1/1,000 people who undergo sequencing are super responders. I suspect this Fermi estimate is not far off.

How Should We Assess Precision Oncology?

Precision oncology meets the two major criteria that warrant a randomized controlled trial (RCT). First, it is an intervention postulated to benefit patients. Second, it offers a marginal to modest effect size (see glossary) at best. The rational way to test it is with an RCT. Moreover, one has even been performed. The SHIVA randomized trial assigned patients with molecular alternations in one of three pathways to a drug matched to that pathway (11 drugs available) or a physician's choice of treatment without knowledge of the mutation. Among 195 people included in the study, there was no difference in the median progression-free survival between the two treatment strategies.[15] There is at least one ongoing RCT, entitled IMPACT-2.

There are some proponents of precision oncology who prefer retrospective observational studies (see glossary). As we will see in chapter 9, there are pitfalls to such an approach. These studies compare patients for whom mutations were found and received targeted drugs against those for whom there were no targeted drugs for their mutations.[16,17] However, these two groups of patients are fundamentally different. One is filled with people who have mutations where drugs are available, and the other is filled with people who have mutations where there are no drugs that target them. These un-drugable mutations are probably that way for a reason—they are probably nasty, bad biology mutations like loss of *p53* or activating *Ras* mutations. If you don't know what those are, you can ignore that digression. But, the bottom line is you cannot compare people with one set of mutations taking drugs for them against a group of patients with different mutations entirely. That is essentially comparing apples to oranges.

What Do We Need Now?

I think it may someday be possible that genetic sequencing and paired therapy will be superior to current standards in all tumor types, but based on all the information we have at present, that day is not today. In the meantime, commercial testing agencies and academic medical centers are not marketing genetic sequencing like a test in need of validation. They are marketing it as if it was a miracle. I find this to be little better than the selling of snake oil to cancer patients. It is preying upon the sick by creating the illusion that you can make them better off without knowing if that is true. To understand the effects precision medicine has on clinical endpoints, and move it into the realm of evidence-based medicine, we need a randomized trial. I suggest one of the two randomized trials (fig. 8.1).

Observational research on precision oncology inadvertently provides a path forward for RCTs. Using the estimates postulated by these studies, I designed the sample size needed for an RCT. It is worth noting a few things. First, the benefits of precision oncology, even using upwardly biased observational data, are still far less than what we would want for patients. An improvement in survival from 8.9 to 10.1 months if you get sequenced? Those 1.2 months would put precision oncology alongside the most mediocre cancer drugs, and that is if the

Version 1   Version 2

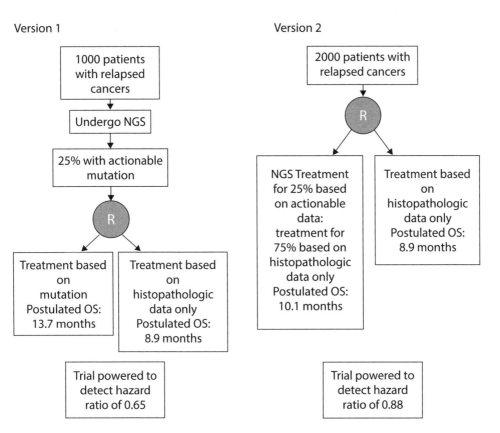

Figure 8.1. Two proposals for randomized trials of the precision oncology strategy. Used with permission by Oxford University Press *Annals of Oncology.*

trial is successful. The second thing to note is just 1/100th of the patients who have undergone sequencing could be used to test the strategy.

Yet, no matter the result, trials examining the effectiveness of these strategies have high value to patients and society. There is continued spending on these strategies without clear evidence they help people. The cost of settling the question pales in comparison to the snowballing price of the therapy. Even though some proponents have ossified in their pro-precision oncology stance (helped by financial conflict of interest), many doctors still keep an open mind and would change their view. For these reasons, my proposed randomized trial is a good use of resources.

Conclusion

Precision oncology—meaning broad sequencing in all people with cancer—is just another hypothesis. It is a seductive one. What patient or doctor wouldn't want a therapy tailored uniquely to them? But the reality is that most patients don't match, most patients don't respond, some patients would get different drugs if they used different tests, most responses don't last, and, on average, whether the strategy is superior to alternatives remains uncertain. Perhaps someday we will see the success of precision oncology strategies. But the only way to know for sure would be a simple randomized trial. Precision oncology is a hypothesis in need of appraisal, but that realistic conclusion is one that rubs many people the wrong way.

PART III HOW TO INTERPRET CANCER EVIDENCE AND TRIALS

[NINE]

Study Design 201

One only has to review the graveyard of discarded therapies to discover how many patients have benefited from being randomly assigned to a control group.
Dr. Thomas Chalmers

W E CAN'T get too far in our understanding of cancer policy without having a grasp of the terminology and concepts relating to cancer trials. I call this Study Design 201. Adam Cifu and I wrote Study Design 101, which appears as chapter 9 of our book, *Ending Medical Reversal: Improving Outcomes, Saving Lives.* Here, I focus on the designs used to study cancer therapies.

Two of the most common study designs are observational studies and randomized controlled trials. For randomized trials, there are some unique design features that are almost exclusive to cancer medicine. The major virtue of randomization is put in context by comparing it to and contrasting it with two other common types of studies in cancer.

Before we get started, let's think back to the clinician and researcher. In *Ending Medical Reversal,* we contrast two different types of scientists. First, are researchers. These are folks who care about fundamental questions about why the world works the way it does. Next are clinicians. These are folks seeking practical answers to decisions they face in the clinic, in the process of taking care of people with cancer.

There are many questions a researcher may have, and the right study design is the one suited to answer that particular question. You may wonder: Why does cancer exist? What percent is due to environmental causes versus genetic causes? Why are some tissues in the body affected more often than others? Some of these questions are incredibly challenging, and I don't have the answer to many of them. But, the most common question faced by those who take care of people with cancer—the most relevant and pertinent question for the clinician—is: will this pill, procedure, surgery, or radiation course help? Should I offer this to my patient? In this chapter, we will focus on these questions. When it comes to assessing whether doing something will make people better off, here is what you need to know.

Going Nuts

In May of 2017, a story broke in the national news. Headlines read, "Are Nuts Good Medicine for Colon Cancer Survivors?"[1] And "Eating Tree Nuts May Cut Risk That Colon Cancer Will Return."[2]

Researchers found that colon cancer patients who had a localized cancer removed had a reduction in their risk of cancer recurrence if they ate more than 2 oz. of nuts a day.

Before I tell you why this was nuts, you should know something about the drugs proven to reduce the risk of colon cancer recurrence in randomized trials and those that haven't. Drugs that lower cancer recurrence have something in common.

In a meta-analysis, the chemotherapy drug 5-FU reduces death by 22% (from 83% to 78%) for patients with colon cancer who have undergone surgery.[3] Adding oxaliplatin, another chemotherapy drug, further reduces the risk of recurrence (in stage 3 cancer) by 20% and death by 16%.[4] Bevacizumab, which arguably has a small benefit in the metastatic setting, failed in at least three trials in the adjuvant setting.[5-8] Irinotecan, a useful drug in the metastatic setting, also failed to reduce risk in the adjuvant setting,[9-11] as did cetuximab, which offers a small survival advantage in the metastatic setting.[12,13]

So what is the take-home lesson? Simply working in the metastatic setting is no assurance a drug will work in the adjuvant setting, but I am aware of no substance on earth that reduces risk in the adjuvant setting that doesn't shrink tumors in the metastatic one.

Now, let's turn to nuts. Does eating 2 oz. of tree nuts shrink metastatic cancer? Absolutely not. If this were the case, we would find in the literature anecdotal reports of feeling great after two fistfuls of almonds, but there is no such report. It is not even plausible a benign substance like nuts would result in the death of cancer cells. At the outset, what does that tell you about the possibility that nuts are beneficial after we surgically remove colon cancer, arguably a higher biological hurdle?

Now, what did researchers find? Eating 2 oz. of nuts resulted in a 42% lower risk of cancer coming back and a 57% lower risk of death.[1]

Does that make sense? First, not only do nuts lower the risk of cancer returning, they have an even bigger effect on death! Even if you believed nuts prevented cancer from coming back that isn't enough to explain the full survival gain. You need to postulate another 15% benefit on top!

Second, the value of nuts—the benefit provided—appears to surpass all chemotherapy drugs. Nuts seem to be the single greatest intervention to reduce colon cancer recurrence. But "this benefit was limited to tree nuts such as Brazil nuts, cashews, pecans, walnuts and pistachios, said [the] lead researcher," who was a clinical fellow at Harvard.[1] As if that makes it more plausible, not less.

Okay, what really happened? People who eat 2 oz. of tree nuts (but not peanuts) per day are unique people, who are going to do better than the average person. Not only are they rich enough to afford their tree nut habit, but they have the time and luxury of being able to stock their cabinets with tree nuts; they have the presence of mind to include these tree nuts in their daily routine. I am not sure that, when I was a medical student, resident, and fellow, I could afford the tree nuts; now, as a physician, I can support a 2 oz. per–day tree nut habit, but I don't have the time and energy to regularly incorporate these into my diet.

What sort of people do? These are very special people, who are socioeconomically well-off, and have the time and energy to focus on their health. Perhaps these people had their cancer discovered slightly sooner than those who do not eat tree nuts.* Perhaps these well-off

---

* This can happen despite the fact they are both the same stage, as a stage is a category with some room within it. Like an income bracket. Just because you share a bracket, doesn't mean you have the same income.

patients have different biology in their tumors. Perhaps they take part in other health behaviors that lowers their risk.

Whatever the reason, these are unique people, and they are not comparable to the others. Moreover, the fact survival benefit is larger than cancer recurrence benefit is actually more compatible with the idea that there is something about the people, and not the nuts, that is making them better off. After all, reduction in cancer still doesn't explain the full degree to which they are better-off.

But the real lesson here is that researchers can make mistakes. Out of a desire for publicity, or professional acclaim, or perhaps because they simply don't know better, Harvard researchers can attach their name to something that is almost certainly false.[14,15]

Vibration of Effects

There is a deeper problem with research like this. It is the problem of multiplicity—or the number of times you test something. We will soon see that one of the virtues of randomized trials is that they limit multiplicity. On the other end of the spectrum are studies like this: nutritional epidemiologic studies. When it comes to nuts or berries or wine or coffee, we have very few—nearly no—randomized trials. All of our studies are observational studies. The problem with observational studies is twofold. First, there are differences between the people who partake and choose not to partake in these studies. People who eat 2 oz. of tree nuts a day are different from those who don't. The second problem is there are very few limits to the sheer number of times the same or similar analyses are performed.

Consider tea, coffee, metformin, statins, aspirin, vitamin E—it would not be surprising to open the newspaper and read that vitamin E increases all-cause mortality. Perhaps the next week, it may read, vitamin E decreases it! The same is true in studies for all these common nutritional exposures. Coffee is great for you. Now it's poison. It is clear, the news perennially flip flops on these topics.

In 2015, Chirag Patel and colleagues sought to explain why there are so many contradicting nutritional studies.[16] To understand their paper, you have to understand how researchers study these exposures. Because there are no large trials randomizing people to recommendations for drinking more or less coffee, researchers use observational datasets. One popular and widely available dataset is called NHANES (National Health and Nutrition Examination Survey). A lot of researchers have access to it and can run analyses with it, especially for hot questions. To do so, they go back in time and compare people who had the exposure (for instance, coffee) against those who did not. They look to see if one group experienced the event—death or developing cancer or anything you wish—more or less often than the other group. And the final thing they do is adjust for pertinent variables. They adjust for age, or sex, or socioeconomic factors. They may adjust for race or family history of heart disease, for example. They adjust for these factors because the researchers want to ask: holding all else constant, does coffee consumption have anything to do with how long you live?

The insight of Patel and colleagues was to study what happens when you consider multiplicity. What if a researcher in Portland adjusts for age and sex? A researcher in Toronto adjusts for age, sex, and socioeconomic factors.* A researcher in Atlanta adjusts for four other factors. One in Boston adjusts for six.

Patel and colleagues realized that even if individual researchers adjust for only a handful of factors, or combinations, others might adjust for different handfuls. Across the world, researchers may effectively be testing the hypothesis with nearly all possible sets of variables being adjusted for. They decided to simulate this.

They picked several popular nutritional variables and tested their effect on mortality. Using a computer, they adjusted for all possible combinations of 13 commonly used adjustment factors (like, age, race, sex, socioeconomic factors, and so on). The authors found that 31% of things they studied could get both positive or negative associations with mortality, simply by picking different factors to adjust for. Something like vitamin E could protect you or lead to your early death, depending on what else about your life is taken into consideration in the model. They called this *vibration of effects.*

* Maybe they care about these factors more in Canada.

The vibration of effects is the deep problem with observational research. The majority of relationships of common exposures and common outcomes (like cancer) are probably neutral—the food does not markedly change one's long-term risk of death. And, that makes sense. After all, is it really plausible that a cup of coffee or tea twice a day has anything to do with how long you live? Or one extra serving of carrots? The truth is that most common exposures have no major contribution to living longer. At the same time, if many investigators are pursuing the idea and incentivized by the fact that splashy findings get your name out there, the end result might be a system similar to what we have: where findings are constantly touted and often contradict each other. Each published article is just the significant tip of a very large uninteresting iceberg.

When Observational Studies Are Followed by Randomized Controlled Trials

Consider what happens when observational studies and RCTs are performed on the same topic. Observational studies cannot be performed for drugs that are not FDA approved and not on the market because there would be no participants to observe taking said drugs. They can, however, be performed for drugs already approved for at least one purpose, even if it is not the purpose the investigators wish to study. This is due to the fact that once a drug is for sale, doctors often use them for purposes beyond what they are approved for. This is called off-label use. Moreover, the 21st Century Cures Bill, a piece of federal legislation signed at the end of the Obama administration, actually permits the FDA to use such studies for approval. By the end of this chapter, you can decide for yourself if you think that is a good idea.

Take bevacizumab, a cancer drug I discussed in chapters 1 and 2. As you may recall, bevacizumab was approved in combination with chemotherapy in the initial treatment of metastatic colon disease. Its widespread use, however, could be questioned by some, because in practice the drug was combined with a different chemotherapy for which we had negative trial results. Yet, in the mid-2000s, researchers were concerned about a different question. At that time, there were no data on whether bevacizumab use is effective in patients whose cancer inevitably progressed on the initial bevacizumab + chemotherapy regimen. The standard paradigm was to switch to a different chemotherapy, but should the bevacizumab be stopped or continued?

In 2008, an observational study tried to answer this question. The study was called BRiTE,[17] which stood for Bevacizumab Regimens: Investigation of Treatment Effects and Safety.* BRiTE did something simple. It compared three groups of patients: (1) those who did not get any treatment after the first progression (these patients are likely very ill); (2) those who got more chemotherapy without continuing bevacizumab; and (3) those who got more chemotherapy plus bevacizumab. The results were dramatic. The median survival was 12.6 months for patients who got nothing (not surprising), 19.9 months for those who got chemotherapy alone, and 31.8 months for those who got chemotherapy and bevacizumab. If you believe BRiTE, bevacizumab improved survival by a whopping 11.9 months. That's nearly a year of improvement—a 60% improvement in survival.** Think back to chapter 1. The average cancer drug has about 2.1 months of benefit. If BRiTE were true, the effect would be staggering.

Randomized Controlled Trials

Fast forward to 2012, when the question of bevacizumab's effectiveness was revisited. While BRiTE was an observational study asking what happened to patients in the real world, ML18147*** was a randomized trial that compared second-line chemotherapy with or with-

* Many people love giving their study a catchy acronym. An astute clinician once noted that six of the seven deadly sins can find a medical trial acronym that fits "CASANOVA, PASTA, MIDAS, SWORD, CADILLAC, PARAGON."[18] There has been no funding for sloth. "These trials are more likely to be cited even after adjusting for multiple factors."[19]
** I hate the use of relative risk (the 60% change noted here), which has rightly been called "lying with statistics." I use it here only to compare it to another relative risk mentioned later in this chapter and not to sell you on the drug.
*** Doesn't that just roll off the tongue. Makes you wish it had a trendy name like AVASTIN4EVER.

out bevacizumab. This study sought to answer the question: what is the value of continuing bevacizumab for patients moving on to the second chemotherapy in metastatic colon cancer? Unlike an observational study, a randomized trial is a formal experiment. Patients are enrolled and do not know what they are getting. They are then randomly assigned, often by a computer program, to one treatment or another. Some patients get the intervention and some don't, and then we compare the results between the two groups.

I alluded to this in chapter 8; there are two prerequisites for a randomized trial. First, there is equipoise for the effect of the intervention. Randomized trials aren't needed for interventions with very large effects. Second, the intervention is something that we hypothesize will benefit patients.

If the intervention is something like wearing a parachute and jumping out of a plane, where death is all but certain without the parachute and survival all but guaranteed with it, then, sure, you can just use common sense. The truth is that there are few medical practices this successful. Almost nothing we do in health care takes survival from 0% to nearly 100%, so the first prerequisite doesn't exclude too many medical interventions.

The second prerequisite is that there needs to be a belief that the intervention has benefit. I am compelled to say this, though it may seem obvious, but randomized trials are not performed for potential harms. No one, besides war criminals, would randomize a person to a harmful intervention. If one thinks exposure to industrial solvents causes cancer, you wouldn't conduct a randomized trial offering people solvents. The same goes for smoking. The same goes for a gunshot wound. Yet, you will find many smart people saying since we didn't do a randomized trial of smoking (a harmful intervention), we can't do a randomized trial of [insert their favorite practice].

However, if you are creative, you can often flip the design of the study to get an answer to your question in an ethical way. For instance, you can't randomize patients to smoking, but you can take heavy smokers who are set in their ways and randomize them to cessation strategies. Randomized trials work well in medicine because most of what we do has a medium effect at best, and all of what we do is trying to make the world a better place.

Now that I have clarified when randomized trials are possible, let's consider their advantages. The first advantage is that the two arms of a randomized trial are balanced in other variables that might affect the outcome. Perhaps patients who take bevacizumab after progression are wealthier (with better insurance) than those who don't take it. Perhaps it's the wealth and the support that it buys and not the bevacizumab responsible for the better outcome. This would not happen if we randomly assigned patients to bevacizumab. In this case, we would expect both groups to have people across the socioeconomic spectrum, and in comparable distributions.

The second benefit of randomized trials is limiting multiplicity. Multiplicity essentially means the number of times you can test something. Because there are added burdens to conducting randomized trials, the total number of times you can test something is limited. These burdens do not exist with observational studies, where you can test as many times as you wish. Multiplicity is the key to the vibration of effects phenomenon we discussed earlier. Ideally, you look for a few randomized trials showing comparable results, but in no case do we have ten thousand on the same topic, and researchers get to cherry pick the one that fits their preconceived belief.

Returning to our question: should bevacizumab be continued upon progression? The ML18147 trial tested the same exact question as the BRiTE study.[20] In the ML18147 trial, patients were all given chemotherapy and randomly assigned to bevacizumab or not. Survival in the patients getting chemotherapy was 9.8 months, compared to 11.2 months in the group getting chemotherapy and bevacizumab. Bevacizumab improved survival 1.4 months, or 14%. Remember, it was nearly 12 months in BRiTE. Why the difference between BRiTE and ML18147?

These two trials illustrate a common problem with observational studies in cancer medicine. There are complex social and biological reasons why some patients and not others receive cancer drugs in the real world. Patients who are physically stronger are often more likely to receive these drugs than those who appear ill or infirm. For this reason, comparing those who got the therapy to those who did not is fraught with problems. In the case of bevacizumab, an 11.9-month benefit became a 1.4-month benefit after confounding influences were minimized by randomization. By doing so, the benefit nearly disappeared. Later, I will give you reasons to doubt even the 1.4-month benefit found in the randomized trial, but let us turn to the final study design in cancer medicine I want to discuss: the historically controlled trial.

Historically Controlled and Uncontrolled Trials

There is a hybrid study design that has certain elements of a retrospective (looking backward in time) study design, using observational data, and a randomized trial. That is the historically controlled trial. A historically controlled trial is an experiment, but unlike a randomized trial, everyone gets the therapy. You essentially compare 70 patients under your care getting the investigational therapy to patients who previously received care but did not receive the investigational therapy.

Consider a fairly common cancer called non-Hodgkin's lymphoma (NHL). Since the 1960s, the standard of care to treat advanced NHL was a combination of three chemotherapy drugs and prednisone called CHOP (cyclophosphamide, doxorubicin, vincristine, prednisone). These drugs produced complete response approximately 45% to 55% of the time and had a long-term disease-free* rate of approximate 30% to 35%.[21]

In the 1980s, many ambitious cancer researchers thought they could improve upon that. At the National Cancer Institute,** then the mecca of global cancer research, researchers pioneered more complicated, multidrug treatments with fancy names like ProMACE-cytaBOM. These combos clearly had more toxicity, but it was believed that they

---

* Some might just say cure rate, but I am very careful not to use that word, for reasons covered in prior chapters.
** Full disclosure: I trained in hematology oncology at the NCI. I have incredibly fond memories of the place.

would save more lives. Also, their names were far more impressive. Say it with me: Pro-Mace-Cy-Ta-Bom!

In 1991, the NCI reported the results of its trial* with ProMACE-cytaBOM.[22] They gave the therapy to 94 patients who had non-Hodgkin's lymphoma. The results were astounding. Eighty-six percent of patients had complete response, and the long-term response appeared to be nearly 69%. These results were simply much better than CHOP did historically, and although some investigators at the NCI expressed caution,[23] ProMACE-cytaBOM was accepted by many as gospel.

An NIH faculty member once told me a story about ProMACE-cytaBOM. In the early 1980s, this person joined the NIH from a prestigious Midwestern hospital. At that time, one of the ProMACE pioneers asked him what he had used, prior to joining the NIH, to treat people with lymphoma. He remarked CHOP. The senior researcher laughed. "Do they still use CHOP there?" he mocked. A decade later he would eat those words.

In 1993, a randomized trial was performed to settle the question.[21] Nearly 900 patients were randomized to CHOP, ProMACE-cytaBOM, or two other promising combinations. The results were surprising. At three years, all groups had approximately a 44% chance of being alive and free of lymphoma. The complete response rate of ProMACE-cytaBOM was 56%—30 percentage points lower than what the NIH had previously reported! Some researchers wondered if the discrepancy was due to dose reductions of the medications in the randomized study, but they looked at this specifically, and the dose was identical to that given at the NCI.

The take-home lessons of ProMACE-cytaBOM are twofold. First, historically controlled studies are notoriously inaccurate. In 1982, three researchers compared historically controlled and randomized trials on *the same clinical question*. They found that 77% of the time histori-

* This was technically part of a randomized trial of 190 patients. The randomization, however, was not against the current standard of care, but two different versions of Pro-MACE therapy. The authors just wanted to perfect the Pro-MACE therapy. Practically speaking, the authors were using the Pro-MACE-cytaBOM arm as a single-arm study. Moreover, there was another, similar study reported by the Southwest Oncology Group a few years before.

cally controlled trials found a therapy beneficial, but this was true in only 20% of randomized trials.[24] The lesson is clear—take historical controlled trials with a grain of salt.

The second lesson is yet another one about response rate. The complete response rate of ProMACE-cytaBOM was 30 points higher in the NCI experience than in the major randomized trial. Is this common? As it turns out, it happens all the time and is another reason to think critically about response rate. Zia and colleagues examined the response rate for the same drugs in the same cancers in both a randomized trial (phase 3 trial) and a prior study (phase 2 trial). They found the response rate was 12.9% higher, on average, in the prior study than in the randomized trial.[25] The NCI experts were right about one thing, ProMACE-cytaBOM is above average in one respect: loss of response rate.

Crossover

There is one special feature that sometimes occurs in cancer randomized trials, which is vital to understand. That feature is called *crossover,* or *unidirectional crossover.*[26,27] Crossover means that, at some point, patients who were assigned to the control arm of a trial (either the established standard of care drug or placebo) are allowed to receive the new drug after they have progressed (fig. 9). Understanding crossover is complicated. In RCTs, there are situations where you want crossover and situations where you don't. Being able to delineate whether crossover is appropriate in various situations means that you understand cancer trials at a high level.[28]

Where Is Crossover Necessary?

If a drug has already shown benefit as the second or third treatment for a cancer, and you want to test whether it should be moved up and used as the first treatment, you need crossover.*

For instance, a randomized trial called Keynote-024 did this cor-

* Some researchers would call this appropriate post-protocol therapy instead of crossover, and that is fair, but the principle stands.

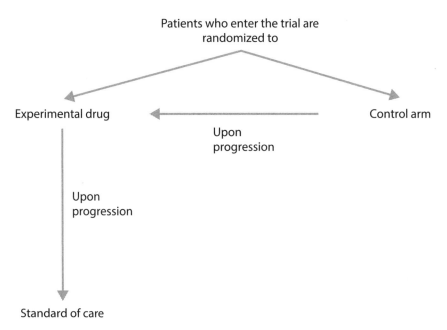

Patients who enter the trial are
randomized to

Experimental drug ⟵ ⟵ Control arm
Upon
progression

Upon
progression

Standard of care

Figure 9.1. Crossover in randomized trials

rectly.[29] The drug pembrolizumab, one of those new immunotherapy agents, had already been shown to be the preferred second therapy for patients with non-small-cell lung cancer and a high expression of PD-L1. (If that sounds like a foreign language, let's just say "shown benefit for a form of lung cancer.") Researchers wanted to know whether it was better to give pembrolizumab as the first-line therapy. Of course, this is a fair question, and to test it fairly you should randomly assign patients to pembro first (the experiment) versus current best practice, which is pembro second. This trial allowed crossover, as it should have, and showed a survival advantage. Doctors can feel confident that for this subtype of lung cancer, pembro first is best.*

At other times, we want crossover, but researchers fail to deliver. This often happens when trials that are meant to inform decisions made in the United States but are conducted in countries whose prac-

---

* Assuming there are no other problems with this trial. So far, I have not seen any, but history has taught me to keep an open mind and avoid final verdicts. For now, however, I do use pembrolizumab in this population.

tice of medicine is different from that in the United States. All randomized trials, by their nature, need comparison or control groups, and those control groups should receive therapies in accordance with the standard of care. Yet some countries, due to limited resources, do not offer the same drugs we would in the United States. By itself, the way these other countries practice medicine isn't necessarily bad. But what this means is that we may remain unsure if the new drug would have the same result were it tested using US standards. For this reason, it may also be reasonable to say to drug companies, "Look, if you want to get regulatory approval in the United States, you have to conduct your trial in—this is going to sound crazy—the United States."

Consider a trial called LATITUDE[30] that sought to "move up" a costly new drug called abiraterone in the treatment of prostate cancer. In the United States, we were already using abiraterone in a more severe disease setting. In the LATITUDE trial, researchers gave the medication much earlier than current practice. The trial showed a survival benefit, and when I read it, I remember thinking, "Okay, that's convincing." But, I had forgotten to double check if patients who were assigned to the control arm received abiraterone after progression as they otherwise should have. Weeks later, when I read the letters to the editor, I learned they had not.

DeBono and colleagues write that "the majority of men in the control groups in the STAMPEDE and LATITUDE trials died without exposure to abiraterone or enzalutamide. Thus, the drugs used in these control groups were inconsistent with current prevailing standards of care. This has implications for the conclusions of the trials and raises questions regarding whether or not there was a benefit for all trial participants."[30]

Boom! You were supposed to allow these patients crossover, but you didn't. That's not just slightly bad; this sort of error entirely invalidates the study and makes drawing conclusions from it useless.

Where Is Crossover Problematic?

There are situations in oncology where having crossover is problematic. This is generally when you have a new drug that has never been proven to work in any context and researchers decide to allow patients to cross over to the unproven treatment. Why would they do this? There are two reasons given, though I cynically think there is a third reason. The first reason is that crossover encourages patients to enroll in the study. Emerson Chen and I found evidence that this was probably not true. These trials enroll at the same speed as trials without crossover.[31] The second reason is that researchers argue it is ethical. With Christine Grady, head of bioethics at the National Institutes of Health, I argued that this is incorrect.[27] Having crossover in these situations makes interpreting overall survival impossible and actually prevents the trial from answering a meaningful question. A trial that cannot answer any meaningful question is itself unethical because it wastes the time of all participants. The third reason is that it makes it much harder for the drug to fail. If you increase survival despite crossover, celebrate. If you don't improve survival, just say it would have been different if not for crossover. Unless the drug has more deaths in the experimental arm, you have a plausible story to tell. Either way you are a winner!

Let me give you one of the great examples of when crossover should not have happened. First, know that cancer therapeutic vaccines are one class of medication that has consistently failed. For decades, not a single vaccine won regulatory approval. Then in 2010, the first vaccine gained approval. It was called sipuleucel-T, or Provenge. It was used in prostate cancer and was designed to get a man's body to fight his own cancer. Interestingly, in the trial that led to its approval, it did not cause a single response. It did not improve progression-free survival. But it did improve overall survival from 21.7 to 25.8 months.[37]

How did it do this? Possibly because it just takes a long time to kick in, and if we could measure the second or third time the cancer progressed it would be slower for patients receiving vaccine. Alternatively, there may be something to crossover that leads to this scenario.

A report by the Agency of Healthcare Research & Quality (AHRQ) makes this argument.[33] The AHRQ points out that the trial of sipuleucel-T had crossover. Patients assigned to the vaccine who had progression received a drug called docetaxel, which had already been proven to extend survival in prostate cancer, but patients assigned to the placebo received the vaccine when they had progression and then docetaxel if they continued to progress. Due to the design of the trial, among patients who progressed, fewer patients in the control arm received docetaxel, the standard of care, compared to patients in the vaccine arm. For this reason, we cannot be sure whether the benefit in the trial is because the vaccine actually helps, or that those in the control group were harmed by being denied a proven therapy or receiving it at a delayed time point. When faced with such uncertainty, the fact that *every other cancer therapeutic vaccine ever pursued* has failed must weigh heavily in the mind.

In 2017, a different prostate cancer therapeutic vaccine (PROSTVAC) failed in a randomized trial of over 1,200 patients.[34] Notably, this trial did not utilize crossover.

Consider one more example of bad crossover. Medullary thyroid cancer (MTC) is a fairly slow-moving cancer. There are some patients whose cancer takes years or decades to progress, even when metastatic.[35] One drug approved to treat metastatic MTC is vandetanib, which improved progression-free survival in a randomized trial with— you guessed it—crossover. Overall survival was not improved.[36] How we do we interpret a trial like this—a trial with inappropriate crossover that failed to show a survival benefit?

It may be tempting to conclude that, had it not been for crossover, the drug would have improved survival, but that is not certain. There are really three possibilities for what might have happened without crossover:

1. The drug actually does improve survival. For obvious reasons, people love to say this. They miss the corollary that must then be true: If the drug improved survival and if it was crossover that masked the improvement, then you don't have to give the drug right away to see improvement. You can wait to give the drug. You can give it second line.
2. The drug actually worsens survival. Just as crossover can mask a benefit, it can also mask harm. In the case of vandetanib, the

original drug label warned that the agent could cause sudden death from cardiac reasons or death from lung toxicity.[37,38] Imagine if the gains in progression are offset by these deaths. Without crossover and enough time, the drug may actually increase death, but then crossover is implemented and hides the harm. This is another possibility of crossover's effect.

3. The drug has no effect on survival. Whatever gains come from slowed cancer progression are offset by toxicity. All of these three are possible interpretations of a trial like the one of vandetanib.

What have we learned? Crossover is absolutely mandatory when you are asking whether an effective drug should be moved earlier in treatment. Crossover is devastating if it takes places in the first or only trial that seeks to establish the efficacy of a novel compound. Disambiguating these instances takes work, and there are errors of both sorts: crossover used when it is not necessary or not used when it is a must.

Sample Size and Multiplicity

I want to end this chapter with a discussion of two relatively recent problems with randomized trials in oncology. The first is sample size and the second is multiplicity. They both work together to justify ineffective or marginal drugs.

In an analysis of randomized trials in cancer medicine over time, Kay and colleagues found that the number of patients randomized has steadily increased over time.[39] While large sample sizes are a good thing, making for more precise estimates of effect, they have also allowed cancer trials to detect statistically significant but clinically irrelevant differences in survival. For instance, erlotinib in pancreatic cancer was tested in a trial of over 500 patients. This trial was able to find a statistically significant 10–11 day improvement in median survival.[40] This is a benefit that simply is not good enough for patients. Interestingly, the increasing number of participants in studies goes hand in hand with increased industry sponsorship of these trials, which I would argue is a consequence of the current incentive structure. Pharmaceutical companies stand to make billions of dollars from statistically significant but marginal benefits. Even though running these huge trials is costly (more to come on that), the amount of money on the table is so large and the temptation to conduct megatrials chasing trivialities is too great to ignore.

If that is sample size, what is multiplicity? Multiplicity refers to the number of times you test something. If one tests a blue sugar pill against a white one 20 times and uses a p-value of 0.05 (one-tailed) as the threshold of significance, there is nearly a two-thirds chance of the blue pill winning just once. This is multiplicity. When one tests something many, many times, there is a chance that some trials, by chance alone, will be positive. In recent years, there have been calls to take this seriously. Kimmelman and colleagues argue that drugs are best considered at the portfolio level, in light of all the trials that are being conducted.[41] In other words, we have to interpret the results of an *individual* trial in light of all of the trials run on that subject or with that agent.

Consider the PD1 antibody drugs, or immunotherapy drugs, that are often in the news. There are 20 different drugs being studied in 803 trials, with up to 150,000 patients enrolled as of 2016, for this one set of drugs.[42] When we read a single positive finding, should we be thinking of the broader set of trials being run? The answer is almost certainly yes.

My colleagues and I tried to apply this concept to the drug I told you about before—bevacizumab. Bevacizumab has been tested in at least 48 randomized trials.[15] If you look at those trials individually, 30 (64%) report significant PFS gains, and 7 (15%) report improvements in overall survival. However, if you adjust for the fact that you just ran 48 trials, and that some of these might be significant by chance alone, just 21 (45%) trials remain significant for PFS gains, and just 1 (2%) for survival. Moreover, there are likely more bevacizumab trials than these. What does this mean? Is it possible that bevacizumab is a drug that can be combined with many regimens that favorably improves the appearance of tumors on scans, while offering little to no survival benefit, and the fact trials sometimes find benefits is little more than an artifact of how many trials there have been? I don't have the answer, but it is a question that I ponder.

In short, once upon a time, randomized trials minimized confounding and limited multiplicity. Today, because so many trials are being run, they may just minimize confounding. This reduces their value, but randomized controlled trials will remain head and shoulders above other methods of assessing causality.

Conclusion

Historically controlled (or uncontrolled) trials, observational studies, and randomized controlled trials are the tools used to decide what cancer therapies are ready for prime time. Simply being a randomized trial does not mean it is a good trial. You have to think about the sample size, effect size, use of crossover, and number of comparable trials. In this chapter, I didn't cover topics like choice of comparator or rules about who is included and excluded, but I will visit these topics in chapter 13. Hopefully someday soon in cancer medicine the majority of new products will be based on well-done randomized trials. In part IV, I will discuss strategies to ensure this happens.

TEN

Principles of Oncology Practice

To see what is in front of one's nose needs a constant struggle.
GEORGE ORWELL

O VER THE years, I have learned fundamental principles of cancer medicine from many expert physicians. Many of these principles are not given in textbooks and are instead part of the implicit curriculum of oncology. In what follows, I try my best to articulate and document these principles. Some of what follows is my opinion, but far more of it is the unspoken opinion of others who have cared for cancer patients for years. In recent years, however, with new, costly, heavily marketed drugs, I fear these principles are being forgotten.

Adjuvant versus Metastatic versus Refractory

A major distinction in cancer medicine, which I introduced in chapter 2 is the difference between adjuvant drugs and metastatic drugs. To refresh, adjuvant treatment refers to drugs given after a tumor has been cut out entirely and when there is no measurable cancer on a CT scan or other conventional way of testing. Metastatic treatment refers to drugs given when a tumor has already escaped the tissue where it began (a lung cancer spread to the kidney, for instance), and surgery is not an option. Typically, for most solid cancers, the metastatic setting is synonymous with a lethal or terminal cancer. There are many other nuances here when it comes to blood-based cancers or lymphomas, but I am speaking broadly about solid cancers, which are the most common malignancies.

Within the metastatic setting, there is something called line of therapy. First-line therapy means the very first thing with which we treat a patient. Second line is reserved for people whose cancer gets worse (bigger usually) on first-line therapy. Third and fourth lines may then follow. Patients who get many lines of therapy are actually not those with the worst cancer. They often have slow-growing tumors that allow them to live long enough to receive those drugs. People with really bad cancers often have rapid tumor growth and die during first- or second-line therapy or, sometimes, even before they start treatment.

No matter what the setting, the goal of any treatment in medicine is the same: to allow patients, on average, to live longer or better lives. However, there are some key differences between adjuvant drugs and metastatic drugs. Adjuvant drugs are given to patients in whom there is no detectable disease. Some may already be cured of their cancer, but others are destined to have cancer relapse (metastatic cancer), but we don't know who is who. A drug given in the adjuvant setting has a tall task. It has to eradicate microscopic disease in those destined for it to recur, while offering a toxicity profile favorable enough that it does not harm those already cured. The benefits must outweigh harms across all patients. Adjuvant drugs often work better in riskier patients (among those with higher rates of recurrence) and very toxic drugs often don't stand a chance in the adjuvant setting, as you can imagine. In the adjuvant setting, it usually is not enough to delay recurrence or slow tumor growth. You usually need to eradicate the cancer to show a benefit.

In the metastatic setting, the goal remains the same, and more drugs achieve the goal. Typically, a drug merely has to shrink cancer or slow its growth for some period of time to offer a benefit in the metastatic setting. Biologically, this is far easier than eradicating every last cancer cell and, practically, this means that we should not be surprised to find more drugs that help in the metastatic setting than in the adjuvant setting.

In fact, to my knowledge, every drug that works in the adjuvant setting also works in the metastatic setting, while the reverse is far from true. Many drugs that work in the metastatic setting do nothing of real value in the adjuvant setting. Drugs such as irinotecan in colon cancer,[1] sorafenib in hepatocellular cancer,[2] and bevacizumab in colon cancer[3-6] (prior caveats about bevacizumab aside), have some benefits in the metastatic setting but failed in the adjuvant setting. The same story is true for cetuximab in colon cancer,[7,8] erlotinib in lung cancer,[9] lapatinib in HER2-positive breast cancer,[10,11] and the list goes on.

There is one drug that works in the metastatic setting, with a modest PFS benefit, and does very poorly in the adjuvant setting, that received FDA approval.* That drug is sunitinib in kidney cancer. Sunitinib showed a disease-free survival (DFS) benefit in the adjuvant setting in one trial but not in another and not in a pooled analysis.[12] DFS, of course, is a surrogate endpoint. Most importantly, sunitinib did not improve overall survival and actually worsened quality of life. Patients in the ASSURE clinical trial who started taking a full dose of sunitinib (50 mg per day for the first 28 days of each 6-week cycle) discontinued using the treatment due to adverse events at an overall rate of 44% (193/438), and the overall rate of discontinuation remained high at 34% (65/191), even after ASSURE reduced the starting dose of sunitinib (to reduce toxicity) to 37.5 mg for the first one or two cycles of therapy. Similarly, the S-TRAC trial reported that 28.1% (86/306) of patients receiving sunitinib discontinued treatment because of adverse events.[13,14]

Patients in the adjuvant setting may already be cured with surgery alone. For this reason, a principle of oncology is to be more reluctant to use a therapy in the adjuvant setting versus the metastatic setting in the absence of randomized controlled trial data showing overall survival or quality-of-life benefit. Disease-specific survival is really only a validated surrogate endpoint in colon cancer, lung cancer, and head and neck cancer treated with cytotoxic drugs.[15] Yet, some oncologists violate my principle and use drugs that lack randomized controlled trial data, such as cisplatin and etoposide in fully resected small-cell lung cancer (lacks data), 5-FU or gemcitabine in bile duct cancer (neg-

---

* A sinking bar and more to come on FDA reform in chapter 14.

ative data),[16] or gemcitabine and cisplatin in bladder cancer after surgery (lacks data).

There is a broader point here: generally, in medicine, it is far more justifiable to act based on weak evidence when outcomes are poor, patients are symptomatic, and when there are no better data. Compare the front-line metastatic setting to the second, third, or fourth line. For most tumors, we have randomized trial data supporting the first therapy we use. We have randomized data for the second therapy in many settings, but not all. For the third therapy, rarely do we have randomized data. It is far more reasonable to give a third-line drug based on tumor shrinkage alone than to do so in the front line. It is far more reasonable to give a therapy based on tumor shrinkage to a patient who is symptomatic than one who cannot feel a tumor that is only visible on CT scan.

For those with very small amounts of metastatic disease, who may have had it detected incidentally, meaning they have no symptoms, it is often reasonable to watch the patient closely before initiating treatment. Most of the trials validating front-line therapy studied patients whose cancer presented with some symptom. If cancer is treated, shrinks, and recurs, asymptomatically, a prudent oncologist may watch a patient with scans to decide the right moment to treat the patient.

Putting all this together, one can imagine a continuum of risk and benefit. On one end are patients with early, small, asymptomatic or undetectable disease, and at the other end are patients with advanced, bulky, debilitating cancers. We must demand better evidence for the former than the latter—for the simple reason that we are more likely to do net harm and not improve things for the former than the latter. If we start talking about chemoprevention, the bar must be even higher—proving an overall survival advantage for any average or modestly elevated risk patient who feels healthy* (more to come). We should not forget that treating a patient will certainly bring toxicities and costs. The question is always: do the benefits outweigh those downsides?

---

* I make an exception for ultra-high-risk genetic conditions like *BRCA1* mutations coupled with a strong family history.

Treating until Progression: Does It Make Sense?

I have spent time in this book explaining why progression is an artificial threshold and often correlates poorly with survival. At the same time, many providers use progression as the basis to discontinue therapies or switch therapies. Of course, in these cases, they could be making the same error—using an arbitrary standard to stop a drug. Sometimes, they may be switching too early and other times they may be switching too late. The 2009 RECIST guidelines (that explain what response and progression are) make this point: "Many oncologists in their daily clinical practice follow their patients' malignant disease by means of repeated imaging studies and make decisions about continued therapy on the basis of both objective and symptomatic criteria. It is not intended that these RECIST guidelines play a role in that decision making, except if determined appropriate by the treating oncologist."[17]

Consider the case of sunitinib for metastatic kidney cancer (not adjuvant, but metastatic). It was (at the time of this writing) standard practice to use sunitinib as the initial treatment of metastatic kidney cancer, and, when patients progress, switch to axitinib or pazopanib, a different, albeit similar tyrosine kinase inhibitor. Arguably this is the cancer equivalent of switching from Coke to Pepsi, and led investigators to study the topic, making a few observations.

First, sunitinib inhibits vascular endothelial growth factor (VEGF) signaling, which is nearly an identical mechanism to several other drugs that are used after sunitinib. Second, sunitinib and the other drugs used in this setting improve PFS modestly, and mostly by slowing tumor growth. These authors then created a model of tumor growth and death and argued that continuing sunitinib at progression might further improve outcomes, compared to stopping it at progression in order to switch to another drug.[18] Their reasoning went like this. No drug can halt tumor growth, but all slow tumor growth, but as long as progression is 120% growth—you will eventually progress with any drug. So switching makes sense only if the new drug retards growth more than the old drug, but these researchers felt the data did not support this idea. You would be better off sticking with sunitinib than switching, they argued. Such a claim should not be entirely surprising when the replacement drug is nearly the same as the original treatment. It's like switching brands of coffee between cups. You probably get the same coffee buzz by drinking more of the same, and brewing new coffee instead of pouring from the same pot may be unnecessary.

At other times, progression might be too late to discontinue a drug. Consider a heavily pretreated patient—someone who has already received many drugs in the past. Although many believe that the number of prior therapies is a marker of how sick a patient is, often the reverse is true. These patients are heavily pretreated because they lived long enough to receive so much therapy. Their cancer's biology was so slow that doctors had plenty of time to try out new drugs. It reminds me of the Voltaire quote, "The art of medicine consists in amusing the patient while nature heals." In this case, the drugs may provide little value to the patient while the indolent biology takes its slow course. Imagine, then, putting such a patient on a new drug. There is no tumor shrinkage, but you plan to continue the therapy until progression. Of course, the therapy could just be adding toxicity and providing no benefit.

In short, just as progression is arbitrary and a poor predictor of survival, it may be a bad predictor of when to stop or switch therapies. If it was the stopping point in a well-done randomized trial, then most oncologists would respect it, just as you wouldn't change a cake recipe that works. However, if you are treating someone based on phase 2 data or in a later line of therapy without randomized data or are practicing in a developing nation and have nothing beyond sunitinib in kidney cancer, then one might imagine not being so wedded to a rule that has no fundamental basis. Finally, those who design clinical trials should subject the idea of cancer progression to empirical scrutiny and test alternate starting and stopping strategies for cancer drugs.

Combining Drugs and Extending Treatment

I have made the case that progression-free survival is a surrogate that, more often than not, poorly correlates with survival. Despite this, some oncologists believe that an improvement in progression-free survival can form the basis to change our practice. However, even these advocates of PFS may recognize that there are clearly situations in medicine where progression-free survival is insufficient to change practice. Two of these situations are combining drugs or extending therapy.

Many times in oncology, we use drugs sequentially. In the case of myeloma, we first use a combination of bortezomib, lenalidomide, and dexamethasone (VRD), and later, when the myeloma inevitably returns, we treat with other drugs, including daratumumab (D). Now suppose you want to convince doctors that they should initially use all four drugs (D-VRD) in combination. Well, you have to test D-VRD versus the sequence of the drugs (VRD → D) and show that the upfront combination use of the drugs improves outcomes beyond the sequenced use of the drugs. Looking at progression-free survival makes little sense in this author's opinion because, while the use of more drugs initially may increase the time to progression when progression does happen, you exhaust a drug that you could have saved for a later time.

Take nivolumab and ipilimumab. Both drugs work in melanoma by extending overall survival. It was common practice to prescribe nivolumab then ipilimumab. A study by Larkin and colleagues sought to test whether the combination of the two was better than nivolumab alone or ipilimumab alone.[19] It should be no surprise that PFS was better with the combo, but what do you have reserved for disease once it progresses? The second PFS may even be better with the sequential use of the drugs than with the combination. Moreover, toxicity is worse for the combination. The real question is, which one leads to better survival? Thus far, the combo has not shown superiority in the Larkin study.

To help illustrate the point about combining drugs, imagine you have to go on a long hike and pack a lunch and dinner. You could eat both meals at lunchtime, and if you measure the time until you are hungry, it may be longer with the combination than eating lunch alone, but come dinnertime, you have nothing left to eat, and the sequence of lunch then dinner may be a much better way to ration your meals. I think the point is fairly obvious, but you would be surprised how many oncologists think PFS is all that matters here.

The other scenario where PFS is clearly an insufficient marker is extending a fixed course of therapy, a category that includes maintenance and consolidation therapies (see glossary). There are many situations in oncology where we give four, six, or eight months of therapy and then stop. We wait to see when the disease recurs to decide when to initiate another therapy. These breaks offer many advantages for people with cancer. They allow folks to spend more time at home, recuperate from the toxicity of prior therapy, and have a chance to focus on their life goals. Instead of supporting a break from treatment, companies (not surprisingly) may appear to observers to be seeking market share for new and costly drugs in these situations. Many studies randomize patients to observation or a new $10k/month drug. This isn't necessarily bad science, but the key is the endpoint has to be overall survival. If you are going to accept more toxicity and more therapeutic burden, you can't just delay the time to progression. Moreover, delaying progression is a bit of a triviality. Of course, active anticancer drugs might keep tumors from growing past arbitrary thresholds, but does that result in a longer or happier life?

One analogy for extending therapy is snacking on a long car trip. When you go on a long drive, it is prudent to have a meal, but your goal is to get there quickly. Now imagine two strategies. The first is that you continuously snack on a granola bar, chips, or almonds (you pick). The second is that you wait until you are hungry to stop to eat dinner. Grazing on snacks may certainly delay the time until you stop for a meal but at the price of fumbling with the snack, trying to open it while driving, and getting crumbs everywhere. The reality is that you may need to stop for dinner anyway an hour or two later and ultimately reach your destination at the same time (that's the overall survival of the analogy). Alternatively, the snacking may speed the trip. The question is a testable hypothesis, and one must not assume the answer.

Interestingly, oncology has had some ambivalence on these topics. Trials conducted in the 1990s were interpreted one way—the correct way—while trials conducted in the 2010s have been interpreted another way. Consider this example. When it comes to extending therapy, a famous study from the 1990s showed that a daily chemotherapy drug taken for three months after a fixed therapy improved progression-free, but not overall, survival.[20] This study did not change practice, and no one extended therapy merely to delay progression.

Similarly, a famous study conducted in the 1990s compared breast cancer drug A to drug B to the combination (A+B).[21] It found A+B delayed the time to progression, but it did not result in longer survival or better quality of life over A→B. As such, the trial was widely used to justify the sequence of A→B for years. That paper's 2003 conclusion echoes many of the themes of this book, "Similarly, the inability of increasing response rate and TTF [time to treatment failure] to improve quality of life may reflect the very loose correlation between such standard markers of therapeutic efficacy and quality of life." (See chapters 2 and 3.) It continues, "Indeed, a combination regimen might impair rather than improve quality of life if it induces toxicity disproportionate to response. Until agents with true therapeutic synergy are discovered, sequential chemotherapy represents a reasonable option for patients with metastatic breast cancer."

Now contrast this with nivolumab and ipilimumab, a combination that improves PFS but not OS over nivolumab. This combination has received widespread uptake in melanoma, despite the fact that it adds toxicity and cost, removes a potential salvage therapy, and has not shown survival gain. One potential difference is that in 2018 marketing aimed at persuading doctors to use more therapy may be more effective.

Patients Who Are Asymptomatic

There is an old saying in medicine, "It's hard to make a person who feels fine better off." Of course, this applies primarily to interventions performed on people who don't feel sick: cancer screening, chemoprevention, and the like. There is a hint of truth to this even in the treatment of advanced cancers or metastatic cancers that can be, or often are, asymptomatic, such as smoldering myeloma, follicular lymphoma, slow-growing medullary thyroid cancer, well-differentiated neuroendocrine tumor, and similar malignancies. In my mind, this scenario is a reminder of a principle that suggests that before initiating therapy in these situations, one should ideally have randomized data showing a survival advantage to that or, in the absence of this, one should have evidence that progression has occurred or is imminent. We can debate the second half of the sentence, but the principle is sound: there has to be some reason why you are intervening on an asymptomatic cancer patient. Consider the case of three cancers.

The first is renal cell, or kidney, cancer.[22] It has long been recognized that drugs in kidney cancer are not curative, and there is a small group of patients with low-volume and slow-growing cancers that do not cause symptoms. In 2016, Rini and colleagues found that people with kidney cancer could be followed closely, with providers free to initiate therapy when they felt best. Under this close follow-up scheme, patients had an average of 14.9 months before getting therapy, suggesting that observation is feasible as an initial strategy. Ideally a future study will randomize patients to early initiation of therapy versus later initiation.

Second, with follicular lymphoma, a number of studies support an initial strategy of watchful waiting over therapy for people whose cancers are not causing symptoms or organ damage and are not very large in size.[23-29] In multiple randomized trials comparing early treatment versus waiting to treat, there was no difference in survival—suggesting that early treatment simply increases therapeutic burden and toxicity but does not offer countervailing benefit.

The third example is colon cancer. Two randomized trials have been performed comparing immediate treatment of patients with asymptomatic colon cancer to treatment at the onset of symptoms.[30] Pooled together, these studies found no difference in survival (13.0 versus 11.0 months p = 0.49), and they support the idea of holding off on therapy until symptoms occur.

There are many other examples of asymptomatic early cancer disease states where good physicians watch and wait. In order to change our paradigms here, we need to demonstrate that early treatment improves long-term outcomes. At the same time, we are under increasing pressure to lower the standards and use more costly drugs earlier in disease settings. It's up to the profession to ensure that outcomes take precedence over profits and wishful thinking.

How Hard to Investigate

There is a common challenge encountered in clinical oncology: knowing how much effort to spend in order to work up a diagnosis. How hard should you push to try to biopsy a hard-to-reach abdominal node? How hard should you push to work up nebulous symptoms? A common manifestation of this scenario is when someone asks the question, "Do I need to get a bone marrow biopsy?"

Of course, a novice approaching this conundrum merely asks, "Could the test give me additional information?" A slightly advanced trainee would factor in the likelihood that the test would be positive or negative and ask whether it was worth the effort. A practicing oncologist would ask, "Will it change my management of the patient's care? If the test showed one thing, would I advocate for X, while if it showed another, would I recommend Y?" The best oncologists go beyond this. They consider all of the possible results of the investigation and whether it would change management, and then they factor in what that management change would mean for the patient. If I order a test and get a result and act differently, depending on what the results are, how much better off will the patient be? They consider all of the arms of the decision tree in their mind. They weigh the harms by the potential to add benefit and the probability that the test would push them down a given path. Having performed this mental exercise, they return to the original question and weigh the difficulty and potential harms of the investigation. Only after completing this process do they give their final recommendation. Sometimes it is, "You know what, it will probably be normal, but we really should . . . ," and other times it is, "You know, it is not really worth it for this reason. . . ."

In order to be good at knowing how hard to push, you have to know how you would treat the patient based on the results and the magnitude of the benefit of that intervention. In other words, you have to be highly competent. When you meet an oncologist who does this effortlessly, you stand back in awe. It is medicine practiced well and often with aspiration to be better still in the future.

Chemoprevention

I want to end this chapter with a final principle of cancer medicine that is misunderstood, and that is the role of chemoprevention. An ounce of prevention is worth a pound of cure, or so the saying goes, and indeed many people intuitively believe that it is better to prevent cancer than treat it once it has arrived. I share this intuition and strongly support smoking cessation, an active lifestyle, and other commonsense practices intended to live a longer or better life. However, many people seek out supplements or pills or drugs that might serve as chemical or chemopreventive agents. When it comes to ingesting one of these substances in the hopes of avoiding cancer, I would argue that we have to think broadly.

A healthy person who ingests a substance in the hopes it will prevent cancer is using that as a form of shorthand.[31] What the person might say, when pressed, is, "I want to take a substance that allows me to live longer or better, and hopefully do that by avoiding cancer without any serious secondary side effect or countervailing problem." For instance, a pill that prevented all cancer but guaranteed multiple heart attacks and cardiovascular death would not be what anyone desires or means.

If one takes this principle to its conclusion it means that one wants to prevent cancer in such a way that the cancer benefit translates into an overall benefit on health or quality of life. We don't want a cancer benefit that is eroded by off-target effects (side effects on other organ systems) and, scientifically, the only way to know for sure it is not eroded is for the benefit to carry forward into improved survival or quality of life.

There is another point to be made here. While a healthy person may be reasonably concerned about cancer, if a pill were designed that helps reduce cancer a little, but massively reduces heart attacks and stroke, most reasonable people (who would otherwise be willing to opt for chemoprevention) would take this pill as well. If you are willing to take a pill to prevent cancer so you can live a longer or better life, won't you also consider a pill that prevents stroke or heart attacks to live a longer or better life?

Putting these observations together, I think we don't need *cancer* chemoprevention. We need drugs or agents that improve survival or quality of life in large-scale randomized trials among healthy people. If they operate via preventing cancer—that's great. If they operate via a different mechanism, that's great too. But the relevant test and endpoint should be broad and not necessarily tied to cancer, even if that provided the basic science logic or underpinning for the drug's development.

Conclusion

There are many unspoken rules of cancer medicine, and here I attempt to document a few of them. Many of these principles are commonsense, intuitive, and logical. These rules frame how evidence is developed and trials are interpreted and conducted. It is easy to see how financial and other pressures may wish to change or alter these rules, but we should be cautious in these situations. Ultimately, the purpose of cancer medicine is to use as few drugs as possible for as little time to minimize side effects while simultaneously maximizing survival and quality of life. Often tradeoffs have to be made, but what is concerning are the situations that maximize the use of drugs without increasing benefit. These help profits, not patients.

ELEVEN

Important Trials in Oncology

History is written by the victors.
WINSTON CHURCHILL

Rules are for the guidance of wise men and the obedience of fools.
DOUGLAS BADER

A DISCUSSION of cancer medicine cannot be complete without considering some of the seminal trials that shaped not only oncologic practice but the way in which we conceptualize cancer. In what follows, I will highlight nine drugs and their trials that provide diverse lessons in oncology. I won't spend the majority of this chapter describing the many positive studies in cancer medicine for the simple reason that you could write a several-thousand-page book detailing these. In fact, it exists. It is called *DeVita, Hellman, and Rosenberg's Cancer: Principles and Practice of Oncology*. Instead, I want to highlight quirky or negative trials that change the way we think about cancer and cancer treatment broadly. These are trials that don't get discussed as much, and in my experience, oncologists in training often don't know of their existence. Thinking about these trials can push or challenge the conventional wisdom. Toward the end, I discuss a few positive trials to remind us what we ought to aspire to.

Using a Marker to Guide Chemotherapy

There are many important and long-standing blood cancer markers, and cancer antigen 125 (CA-125) is one of them. This is a marker that is often elevated in the initial diagnosis of ovarian cancer, and for women who have metastatic ovarian cancer and are treated with surgery and chemotherapy, the marker often rises several months before the cancer returns visibly on CT scans or with patient symptoms. Many doctors use the CA-125 in these patients to predict the recurrence of cancer, and some even start treatment at the rise of the marker. In other words, before symptoms arise or cancer appears on scans, the marker may lead to therapy.

In 2009, at the plenary session of the ASCO national conference (aka the big stage), the results of a randomized trial were reported. Researchers compared two strategies of the treatment and management of relapsed ovarian cancer. In one arm, women began treatment when their CA-125 rose to twice the maximum normal value. In the other arm, women were not given information about their CA-125 and were treated only when clinical occurrence was detected (either with imaging or symptoms).[1] This was a clever design testing what some aggressive doctors were doing against what some conservative doctors had been doing. Of course, many followers secretly thought this would prove the value of being aggressive, measuring the marker and treating early.[2]

The first thing the trial showed was that checking a CA-125 accelerated and increased the rate of getting subsequent cancer therapy. Women assigned to acting upon an elevated CA-125 started chemo nearly five months before those in the conservative arm. Nearly 70% started chemo in the first month of being on the trial (fig. 11.1). But the kicker was that even though tumor recurrences were diagnosed *sooner* and appropriate therapy given *earlier,* overall survival was no different (fig. 11.2). Checking patients' CA-125 levels resulted in more chemotherapy being used but also brought side effects. The authors noted that quality of life deteriorated faster for those assigned to early chemotherapy. The authors also noted that there was evidence of "significant disadvantages for . . . emotional, social, and fatigue"–related quality of life scores with early treatment.

The authors understood that the implications of their work extended far beyond ovarian cancer, writing, "Our results challenge the widespread belief that earlier treatment for recurrent cancer must be better,

B Second-line chemotherapy

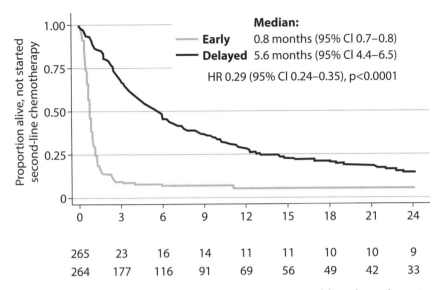

Figure 11.1. Kaplan-Meier plots for time to starting second-line chemotherapy. Early treatment based on increased CA-125 blood levels compared with delayed treatment. Used with permission by the *Lancet*.

A Overall survival

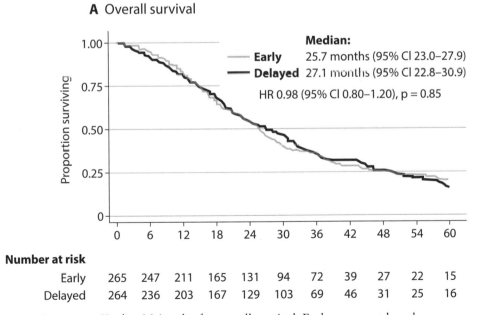

Figure 11.2. Kaplan-Meier plot for overall survival. Early treatment based on increased CA-125 blood level compared with delayed treatment. Used with permission by the *Lancet*.

particularly for cancers for which recurrent disease is disseminated and curative options few."[3] Combine this with the renal cell cancer trials and follicular lymphoma trials from chapter 10, and one might start to see that we need far more trials about the appropriate timing of initiating and reinitiating therapy. For many cancers, particularly those with longer periods of asymptomatic disease preceding progression, it may be better to wait.

Fast-forward seven years from the dissemination of the CA-125 trial results. What do you think happened to medical practice? Absolutely nothing. Esselen and colleagues showed that getting three or more CA-125 tests during surveillance happened to about 86% of women between 2004 and 2009, when we didn't know any better, and to 91% of women between 2010 and 2012, when we certainly did.[4] Some studies hint that we are faster at adopting proven therapies in cancer medicine than getting rid of contradicted ones.[5,6] Regardless of the reason, the CA-125 trial shows just how excessive modern cancer medicine can be. When we know for a fact we harm women by measuring CA-125, we still can't stop.

In news coverage of this story, one expert is quoted describing the phenomenon as "the fundamental attractiveness of testing."[7] Isn't it obvious that more information would be better? The editorial accompanying the paper includes in its title, "Fatal Attraction." And, indeed, the idea that more measurement and earlier treatment is superior in cancer medicine is perhaps one of the core fatal attractions of medicine.

As long as I am on the subject of CA-125, I should mention another use for it. You can probably guess that if you have a blood marker that identifies cancer prior to the onset of symptoms, you can use it to screen for cancer. Of course, CA-125 has been tested as a cancer-screening test, like the PSA for prostate cancer or mammography for breast cancer. Here, the results have also been sobering. In 2011, a randomized trial called the PLCO (short for Prostate, Lung, Colorectal and Ovarian) found that screening with a CA-125 and transvaginal ultrasound failed to reduce deaths from ovarian cancer.[8] A few years later, a European trial found that CA-125 screening (with ultrasound used secondarily) failed to reduce deaths from ovarian cancer.[9] As with many negative trials, the authors instead emphasized a secondary analysis that excluded cases diagnosed in the first round, arguing that there was a hint of benefit. But favoring secondary analyses over primary ones is a bit like drawing the bull's-eye after you shoot. It is clear that more evidence will be needed before this screening is validated. Its benefits will have to be shown to exceed the harms of biopsy, work-up, and overdiagnosis. The lesson here is, for the time being, when it comes to screening, CA-125 also disappoints.

Goldilocks and the Sample Size of Randomized Trials

A few key trials in oncology reaffirm the value of randomized phase 3 trials for drawing definitive conclusions over randomized phase 2 trials. Randomized phase 3 trials are typically larger and use survival as the primary endpoint, as opposed to phase 2 studies, which are correctly viewed as hypothesis generating. Yet, once a phase 2 shows benefit, many act as if the hypothesis is proven, without waiting for confirmatory results. A few key trials make this lesson painfully clear.

Selumetinib is a targeted inhibitor of MAPK kinase (MEK), and in 2012, it was tested in combination with docetaxel against docetaxel alone in advanced lung cancer. The trial showed something remarkable. Survival was extended from 5.2 to 9.4 months, which was not statistically significant, but this was a small, fewer-than-100-person randomized phase 2 trial. Although the primary endpoint was initially PFS, a protocol amendment that authors state occurred "after enrolment was complete and before analysis," switched the endpoint to overall survival.

Leaders called the drug "promising."[10] Yet, just four years later, a 500-person randomized phase 3 trial showed that selumetinib and docetaxel had absolutely no effect on overall survival when compared to docetaxel alone.[11] The authors noted, "The results of this study differ from those observed in a prior smaller randomized phase 2 trial with the same design." The control arm did better, and the experimental arm did worse in the phase 3 trial.

Similarly, iniparib was once considered a promising inhibitor of something called PARP.* In 2011, a phase 2 randomized trial of 123 patients tested whether combining this drug with chemotherapy was superior to chemotherapy alone in a particularly devastating type of breast cancer called triple negative breast cancer.[12] The drug improved response rates by 20 points (from 32% to 52%), progression-free survival from 3.6 to 5.9 months, and overall survival from 7.7 to 12.3 months. All results were statistically significant. The editorialists celebrated the results, "Caveats notwithstanding, these are exciting results presaging improved therapy for an underserved subgroup of patients with breast cancer and, we hope, heralding a new approach of 'setting cancers up for the next blow' by combining cytotoxic chemotherapy with agents directly targeting the DNA-damage response."[12]

A few years later much had changed. Further research cast doubt as to whether iniparib inhibited PARP.[13] It isn't very important to know *how the drug works*. It is more important to have evidence showing *it does work*. A larger randomized trial testing iniparib combined with chemotherapy found that there was absolutely no difference in overall survival. The authors end their paper on iniparib with a wise quote:

> The efficacy results from the phase III study did not confirm the promising results of the phase II study. There were no obvious differences in the patient populations (*BRCA1/2* status data were unavailable) nor in trial designs in the phase II and III studies that could explain these discrepant results. Phase II clinical trial results are hypothesis generating and phase III studies are required to confirm or refute their findings.

A cancer therapeutic vaccine trial reinforces the lesson that phase 2 trials may not steadfastly predict phase 3 results. In the case of PROSTVAC, a vaccine for metastatic prostate cancer that was believed to stimulate the immune system to fight the tumor, a small randomized trial of 125 patients showed a dramatic improvement in overall survival.[14] Yet, the confirmatory phase 3 trial of over 1,000 patients was halted for futility. *Halting for futility* is a statistical phrase that essen-

---

* Short for poly (adenosine diphosphate–ribose) polymerase

tially means that there is an extremely low likelihood that a benefit would ever be shown in further follow-up.[15] In other words, PROSTVAC failed.[16]

The fourth example is the most concerning. This is the drug olaratumab (Latruvo). Not having appreciated that underpowered phase 2 trials can lead to both false positives and false negatives, then FDA commissioner Dr. Scott Gottlieb, testified in front of Congress that survival—not a surrogate endpoint—could be used for accelerated approval.[17] This is a bold expansion of accelerated approval. Remember chapter 3. This pathway is reserved for drugs that improve a surrogate thought "reasonably likely to predict" clinical benefit. Here Dr. Gottlieb was suggesting we expand the category from statistically certain effects on surrogates to statistically uncertain effects on clinical endpoints. This extension would open the floodgates to testing novel compounds in small phase 2 trials, knowing that by chance or randomly getting healthier people on the intervention arm, some will show survival benefit and can slip onto the market, even if they have no evidence of drug activity. Olaratumab was the test case of this strategy. A small trial, not designed for measuring survival, was found to improve survival in people with certain types of sarcoma, from a median of 14.7 to 26.5 months.[18] Based on this, it was approved. And yet, just two years after approval, a larger randomized phase 3 trial found no survival benefit.[19] In the short time it was on market, because it was priced comparable to other cancer drugs, olaratumab generated $500 million in sales for its maker, Eli Lilly.[20] To date, the company has not refunded that money.

Here we have four cases of promising phase 2 trial results contradicted or attenuated by phase 3 trials. So, what happened in these cases? Likely, the difference was due to something called *regression to the mean*. By chance alone, the phase 2 trial was more impressive, and with more data, that effect drifted toward the true effect size, which was no effect. What is interesting is that this phenomenon is likely true for all studies, including small phase 2 trials and large phase 3 trials. We just don't see it with phase 3 trials because these are seldom, if ever, replicated. Moreover, the lesson here should make it clear that Scott Gottlieb and others who wish to expand accelerated approval in this manner are essentially willing to accept massive uncertainty for toxic, costly cancer drugs in exchange for more compounds coming to market at tremendous price.

A final note on sample size: just as clinical trials can be too small, they can also be too large. Recall erlotinib in pancreatic cancer, which was tested in over five hundred people, and found to improve survival by 10 days! Trials that are too large have at least five downsides. First, they are costly. Second, there is an opportunity cost. They enroll patients who could have gone to other trials, answering other important questions. Third, these trials can identify small differences that are statistically significant but not clinically meaningful. Fourth, they can take a longer period of time to enroll and provide results, and fifth, they expose a large number of patients to potentially harmful experimental agents, when fewer could have sufficed. Thus trials are like the tale of Goldilocks: there is a right size.

Responses That Go Nowhere

In chapter 13, I make the case that single agent activity, that is, the ability to shrink tumors, should be the general prerequisite for moving forward in drug development. Not producing responses means a drug is unlikely to greatly benefit patients, but merely having responses is no guarantee of a successful drug. Consider the case of two recent drugs.

Brivanib was once a promising drug for liver cancer. In a study of 55 people who received brivanib, four patients (7%) had responses and 24 (44%) had stable disease.[21] Stable disease only means that the disease had not progressed. When you give a drug to patients who have been chosen for a clinical trial, who are often exceptionally fit, and you don't have a group of patients to compare them against, stable disease is the most useless thing in the world. You have no idea whether stable disease is because the drug slows tumor growth or because you just picked people who are progressing slowly. Regardless, a 7% response rate, although low, was better than some successful drugs in this space. Sorafenib had a 2% response rate and ended up getting approved.[22]

At least four phase 3 trials of brivanib were attempted, further bol-

bolstering the point that drug companies have huge incentive to pursue drugs. The first trial randomized over a thousand patients to either the drug or sorafenib (the current standard of care). In that trial, overall survival was not non-inferior (pardon the double negative).[23] That double negative essentially means overall survival was worse with brivanib, which means do not pass go, do not collect $200, and back to the drawing board. The second trial tested the drug against placebo, among patients whose tumors had progressed on sorafenib. It was also a negative trial, finding no survival benefit.[23] The third trial was like the second trial but in Asian patients, and it was stopped by the company.[24] The fourth trial tested brivanib after local treatment for liver cancer, which ended early after the first three negative trials. The results at that time showed no benefit.[25]

Unlike brivanib, which never made it to the US market, atezolizumab (Tecentriq, Genentech) did receive accelerated approval in May 2016 for second-line bladder cancer. Atezolizumab is one of those new, sexy checkpoint inhibitor drugs that you may have seen a TV commercial about. Atezolizumab got approved based on response rate in a small trial with no control arm. The response rate was modest, just 14.8%,[26] but it was something, and frankly we did not have a lot of options to treat bladder cancer after it progressed on initial therapy.

However, it wasn't long before more sobering results came forward. Proving a drug has a response is proving it has activity against cancer. It is not the same as proving it benefits patients. To prove that a drug benefits patients, you have to show it improves survival or quality of life beyond the best available therapies. To test atezolizumab, a randomized trial was performed. That trial randomized patients to atezolizumab or an older chemotherapy drug picked by the doctor. The primary endpoint was overall survival—a fair endpoint. At the outset, a lot of people, myself included, would say, this is a fairly low bar, and atezolizumab should win. Then, in 2017, we were surprised to learn that atezolizumab failed.[27] Whether or not the FDA will withdraw the drug's approval remains unknown at the time of this writing.

On September 22, 2017, the FDA granted accelerated approval to pembrolizumab, one of those new, shiny immunotherapy drugs, because it could shrink tumors in people with gastric cancer that expressed PDL-1. Specifically, 13.3% of patients had a response with pembrolizumab.[28] Yet, by December of that year, results were not so rosy. Pembrolizumab was unable to improve overall survival when tested against paclitaxel, an older drug.[29] In my memory, it was perhaps the shortest time from an approval based on response rate to a press release of a negative randomized trial. Since it was so fast, I had to ask, "Why didn't the FDA simply wait a few months for these results before making their decision?"

In 2018, the FDA surpassed this strange behavior. On August 16, 2018, the FDA gave an accelerated approval to nivolumab as a single agent for relapsed small-cell lung cancer based on a 12% response rate.[30] What made the approval bizarre was that these results had been more or less known for two years, initially reported in 2016.[31] So while we can debate whether a 12% response rate justifies an accelerated approval, if you think it does, why wait two years? Then, on October 12, 2018 (just two months later), Bristol-Myers Squibb announced that nivolumab failed to improve survival in a randomized trial against chemotherapy for people with relapsed cancer.[32] Although the approval was in the third line, and the randomized trial in the second line, postmarketing commitments in oncology are often customarily in the preceding line. The bottom line here is that two-year-old data were used for an accelerated approval only to be contradicted by a randomized trial two months later. This seems to be bizarre drug regulation.

In 2019, Jennifer Gill and I[33] analyzed all checkpoint inhibitors given accelerated approved on the basis of response rate, and found that 5/31 (16%) failed to improve survival in confirmatory testing. In every one of these cases, the FDA has yet to act, and all continue to hold marketing authorization (at the time of this writing). The social contract of accelerated approval appears to be broken. It is one thing to usher promising drugs to the market based on response rate—we can debate the pros and cons of that; but, it is quite another thing to take no action when that response rate cannot translate into improved survival or quality of life. That appears to be abdicating one's duty.

Before, we leave this section, I have to provide one more example.

This is the case of a drug with a dramatic response rate: more than 60%. And yet, this drug failed to improve survival in multiple studies and was later withdrawn from the US market. That drug is Iodine 131-tositumomab.[34] A long and complicated name, and it is a complicated drug. It is an antibody that binds to cancer cells and delivers a dose of radioactive isotope. Oncologists call such a drug a radioantibody conjugate. In 2003, the drug gained FDA approval with a 68% response rate in relapsed lymphoma. It remained on the market for 10 years before the company voluntarily withdrew the product. Over time, randomized trials emerged that showed the drug did not improve survival in two settings, and the company had no other plans to deliver further proof of benefit. I-131-tositumomab shows the painful lesson that even high response rate is not an assurance a new drug is superior to drugs already on the market.

Nearly All Drugs Benefit People on Average

In 2004, the FDA approved cetuximab for colon cancer, based upon response rate. Cetuximab is an antibody directed against epidermal growth factor receptor (EGFR), which is a protein found to be over-expressed on certain cancer cells that promotes their reproduction and growth.[35] In 2007, a group of Canadian researchers found that cetuximab improved survival when compared to supportive care alone, but the benefit was very small, improving survival from 4.6 months to 6.1 months.[36] That 1.5-month benefit is disappointing, given the drug's side effects, including an often devastating rash.

In 2008, at the plenary session at ASCO, the large international cancer conference,[1] researchers reported a striking observation. They noticed that there seemed to be two groups of patients in the study. Those who benefit from cetuximab had a normal gene called *Ras*, and those who did not benefit had a mutated *Ras* gene. If you had a normal *Ras*, cetuximab improved survival by five months, but it did nothing in those with mutated *Ras*. In the years that followed, we have learned more genetic mutations that identify patients in whom the drug adds no benefit.

The lesson of *Ras* is that, as a general rule in medicine, drugs benefit patients on average. For a group of patients, this drug may improve outcomes, but no one can say for sure that any one patient will benefit or be harmed by a drug, or by how much. All our knowledge about drugs concerns groups of people. Cetuximab worked in all patients on average, and only with time did we find two groups. For one group, it appeared to offer no benefit. For the other group, it appeared to offer a larger benefit, but again *on average*.

Some people point out that just because a drug did or did not work in a randomized trial, it may or may not work for an individual patient. That's technically true, but randomized trials ask the pertinent question: in a given set of patients, do people do better on average with or without treatment? If your RCT is negative, you might say, well there is a subgroup of people in there who would benefit—perhaps with normal *Ras* or some other gene. I don't know yet. But until you isolate that factor and prove the treatment works in this subgroup of patients, it is all speculation. For now, you still don't have a way to find people who benefit, on average. Similarly, if your RCT is positive, that does not mean that everyone in the study benefits. Perhaps a subgroup does not. Yet, by practicing this way, we make the world better on average. Perhaps that is as good as we can do.

The case of cetuximab is the story of a drug that worked (a small bit) in all patients, but that benefit was later found to be driven by only a subgroup. Perhaps in the future we will continue to refine the group that derives benefit even more accurately. Looking for markers (like *Ras*) to identify which patients do not benefit has huge clinical importance. After all, it allows us to spare the toxicity, cost, and inconvenience of cancer drugs from patients who do not benefit from them. Yet, the incentive to look for these factors is limited in the current system. The industry has the incentive to get drugs approved based on the least amount of benefit in the broadest possible population, because this gives them the largest market share. Isolating smaller groups of patients who benefit more greatly from those who do not only limits their sales. As such, one of the major needs for federal funding of research is to do this sort of work.

Non-Inferiority Trials

Non-inferiority trials are a special type of study design that is gaining traction in oncology. In a non-inferiority trial, a new drug does not need to show it is better than an old drug, it just needs shows it is not much worse. Non-inferiority trials are meant to exclude the possibility that a drug is much worse than an older drug.

You probably have a bunch of questions right now. What do we mean by "much worse"? Well, before the trial is run, we specify the difference that would be considered unacceptable, and if the new drug's effect falls within this difference, we consider it acceptable. This difference is called the delta, or margin (more to come on that topic).

Next, you may wonder why on earth anyone would run a non-inferiority trial. Non-inferiority trials should only be run for drugs that are either (1) cheaper, (2) more convenient, or (3) less toxic than older ones. After all, if you are willing to accept the possibility that it is worse than the older drug (but not much worse), you have to have some alternative benefit that would justify the potential loss of efficacy.

Now back to the margin. Several years ago, my colleagues and I examined 17 non-inferiority trials in oncology and found that eight (47%) essentially arbitrarily chose a margin.[37] One trial said the margin was chosen "according to medical judgment of a clinically appropriate and acceptable margin."[38] Let me translate that: "it sounded about right to us." Our findings were confirmed in a larger analysis by Aberegg and colleagues[39] on non-inferiority trials across medicine (not just oncology). Aberegg found that 58% of margins provided no good reason why they were chosen, and another 17% were vague. Alyson Haslam, Jennifer Gill, and I replicated this analysis for oncology trials. We looked across four years of trials in high-impact journals and found that 68% did not justify the margin. Non-inferiority margins are like parallel parking spaces. It takes a skillful driver or a good drug to fit in a tight margin, but even the worst driver or drug can find a way to park on an empty city block. In fact, many non-inferiority margins are ridiculously large, a condition that essentially guarantees non-inferiority. In another study, Flacco and colleagues found that 55 of 57 industry-funded non-inferiority trials got desired results.[40] If non-inferiority trials deliver the desired result 96% of the time, as in this case, then we really have to ask ourselves why they are being performed.

What about alternate benefits? How often are drugs really cheaper, or less toxic, or more convenient? Aberegg and colleagues found in their broad review that 11% of the time a reader could not deduce any such benefit, and only 70% of the time did the study specifically state one. We found similarly that 28% of oncology non-inferiority trials did not give a reason. Consider a few examples of non-inferiority trials in oncology.

Lenvatinib was recently found to be non-inferior to sorafenib in liver cancer.[41] Remember chapter 1? Sorafenib was the first FDA-approved therapy in unresectable, or metastatic, liver cancer, based on a marginal benefit in a randomized trial. In the real world, outcomes were far worse than the trial, and in a propensity score–matched analysis there was no benefit. Lenvatinib is a drug that costs more than sorafenib and offers similar toxicity and convenience. In other words, it has no real alternative benefit to justify a non-inferiority design. Of course, that did not stop the sponsor.

The maker of lenvatinib, Eisai, tested whether the drug was non-inferior to sorafenib. Specifically, it asked if it was 60% as good as sorafenib. No justification for that number was provided. Why 60% and not 50% or 70%? Of course, sorafenib is not a great drug. So here we are testing to see if a newer, costlier drug is 60% as good as a drug that wasn't that good to begin with—it defies common sense. Lenvatinib turned out to meet this low bar, but the tragedy is that 954 patients with a lethal cancer were randomized to this trial, which does not advance care for patients with this condition and only serves to further the market interests of one company.

Now consider the case of pazopanib in renal cell cancer.[42] In a non-inferiority trial against sunitinib, the makers of pazopanib asked if the drug was no worse than a hazard ratio of 1.25. In our survey of oncology trials,[37] we found hazard ratios were deemed non-inferior as high as 1.43. It's worth remembering that a superior drug has a hazard ratio well below 1. Instead, when it comes to non-inferiority, we have drugs that could be markedly worse than their comparator, and some probably are.

Interestingly the authors of the pazopanib-versus-sunitinib study conclude that "quality-of-life profiles favor pazopanib." And yet, a higher proportion of patients discontinued pazopanib (24%) than sunitinib (20%) for adverse events during the trial. Of course, will it come as any surprise that the makers of pazopanib, not sunitinib, funded the study?

The bottom line about non-inferiority trials is they are fine for drugs that are cheaper, less toxic, and more convenient, as long as you pick a conservative margin that ensures patients get most of the benefit of the drug. Sadly, this doesn't appear to happen very often. Instead, and especially in cancer medicine, we see drugs non-inferior to marginal drugs, with permissive margins, that are equally cumbersome and toxic. One fears that this is yet another example of policy favoring profits over patients.

What We Ought to Aim For

Let me end this chapter with just a few examples of what we ought to aim for in oncology. What can we aspire to in cancer medicine?

In 2004, the standard therapy for people with multiple myeloma who could not undergo a bone marrow transplant (either because of age or other medical problems) was melphalan with prednisone.[43] A new drug, bortezomib, sought to improve upon this standard treatment and was investigated through a randomized controlled trial. After a median follow-up of 16.3 months, the addition of bortezomib reduced the risk of death from 22% to 13%. In other words, long before the median survival was reached (that is, the point in time where 50% of patients had died), bortezomib showed it was capable of improving overall survival in this setting, an undisputed benefit. Contrary to popular wisdom, this trial shows you need not wait for median survival to be reached for a potent drug to show a survival benefit.

In 1998, the standard treatment for older patients with large-cell lymphoma was a combination of three chemotherapy drugs and prednisone, collectively called CHOP (discussed in chapter 9). A new antibody called rituximab, which targets the lymphoma cell, was developed, but we did not know if it actually provided benefit for patients. A famous study enrolled older patients with large-cell lymphoma (the average age was 69).[44] This was a bold undertaking. Most Americans with cancer are older, yet trials are routinely conducted in age groups far younger, as we have seen. For a trial to actually recruit older patients is truly remarkable and worthy of praise. After just two years of follow-up, again, long before the median survival was reached, the addition of rituximab improved overall survival in patients with this disease from 57% at two years to 70%. At last, after years of tinkering with CHOP and trying to improve it (including ProMACE-cytaBOM) we finally had something better, and significantly so.

The final example of what we ought to aim for relates to treatment for brain tumors. There are many types of brain cancers, and they range in severity from highly curable tumors to those that portend a poor prognosis. A glioblastoma multiforme is one of the poor prognosis cancers, which affected John McCain and Ted Kennedy. A cancer with a more measured prognosis is low-grade glioma. It commonly occurs in adults younger than 40 and is a life-limiting condition, though someone can live with the disease for years.

A randomized trial of approximately 250 patients tested whether adding three chemotherapy drugs (lomustine, procarbazine, and vincristine, or PCV) to radiation could improve outcomes for glioma patients.[45] Long-term follow-up of that appropriately sized study revealed that median survival was extended from 7.8 years to 13.3 years. Adding 5.5 years of life, on average, is the kind of benefit we ought to see more of in oncology. Powering a trial to find benefits of this size reduces sample size and may even make trials more feasible and useful.

Conclusion

In this chapter, we have explored some examples of important trials in oncology that not only shape our practice but also how we ought to conceptualize cancer medicine. We have seen that valid markers of cancer progression may allow us to give chemotherapy sooner, such as the case with CA-125 for ovarian cancer, but that only delivers net harm to patients. We have seen that randomized phase 2 trials not powered or designed to assess survival can lead to misleading estimates of true overall survival. Yet, in recent years, there has been rhetoric about using these trials as the basis for accelerated approval. That remains an uncertain proposition at best. We have also seen that merely demonstrating a response to therapy is no assurance of having a successful drug. In chapter 13, I talk more about drugs that do not generate responses (spoiler: they generally aren't great); but here, I make the point that merely generating response is not enough to ensure benefit. Finally, I discussed some examples of what we ought to aim for in oncology. To be clear: it is likely idealistic to ask for cures for all cancers, but I think we can ask that new drugs lead to meaningful improvements in survival. Some cancer drugs meet this mark, others don't. The metric of a successful regulatory system is not how many drugs are approved but how many drugs with meaningful benefits are approved. It is time we all started thinking that way.

[TWELVE]

Global Oncology

Close the barn door after the horse has bolted.
ENGLISH PROVERB

OVER THE last few years, I have had the opportunity, and occasionally, the pleasure, to interview applicants for our fellowship program in hematology oncology at OHSU. I've noticed a recurring theme. Many applicants state they want to practice "global oncology." "What's that?" I ask.

Different people mean different things by *global oncology*. Some applicants think global oncology means living and working in a US city while frequently traveling to low- or middle-income nations to administer high-cost (low-value) therapies for a brief period of time until the moment they depart, when care will return to how it had been delivered. Such a view of global oncology is, at best, insulting. Some applicants, however, use the phrase as I do. In my mind, global oncology means investigating strategies or policies to maximally improve cancer outcomes in nations around the world. This matters greatly as low- and middle-income countries have 5% of the global budget for cancer care, but account for 80% of the disability-adjusted life-years lost to cancer.[1]

In this chapter I discuss some of the specific challenges faced globally. The high cost of cancer drugs inflicts some of its greatest damage in low- and middle-income countries. Trials designed to seek US regulatory approval are sometimes performed globally and problematically have used control arms that are beneath the US standard. Finally, I discuss the trials global centers can do instead, trials whose results would be truly transformational at home and around the world.

The High Cost of Cancer Drugs

Research by Dan Goldstein and colleagues investigates the affordability of cancer drugs by nation. It turns out that the United States spends the most on cancer drugs, but given the per capita earnings, cancer drugs are not most unaffordable in the United States. It is in low- and middle-income nations—places like India and China—that drugs are the most unaffordable. Even though the drugs cost less than they do in the United States, the price is high enough to keep them out of reach of most people.[2] When I talk to people who practice extensively in such nations, they tell me that they always take into account what a patient can afford as they devise a treatment plan. A drug that cannot be purchased offers no value to patients.

Different nations have different ways to cope with the problem. The World Health Organization deems some cancer medications as "essential." These are thought to be integral to basic oncologic care, and there are many efforts to ensure these medications are available and affordable around the world. One of the United Nation's Millennium Development Goals is to make sure these medicines are accessible. Other nations have struggled to pay for these drugs, and the story of the United Kingdom's struggle is noteworthy.

The UK Cancer Drug Fund

The United Kingdom does something daring when it comes to medical practices. The nation prioritizes practices based on the cost per quality adjusted life-year (recall chapter 1) and pays for only practices that fall below a threshold. You might think such a policy is foolish or even cruel, but if you step back and reflect, it is a wise decision.

There is only so much money to pay for health care, and by following the United Kingdom's policy, we ensure that we do the most we can with that money. The United Kingdom would prioritize saving 10 lives with a cheap intervention before it saves one life with an incredibly costly one. In other words, the United Kingdom does the most good with each dollar it has. Although it has been criticized regarding its cancer care because it turns down lots of costly, marginal drugs, it makes decisions, on the whole, that benefit its population. And guess what? Its life expectancy is longer than in the United States.[3]

In 2010, under immense political pressure, the United Kingdom created a separate fund to pay for cancer drugs. This fund would be used to pay for drugs that would not otherwise be covered in the UK system, that is, marginal drugs that cost a lot but offered little gain. The United Kingdom would negotiate a confidential discount with the drug company, which would provide the drugs to people with cancer. While the proposal seems to make sense, it practically means that money used for the cancer drug fund (CDF) would be paying for drugs that cost a lot and delivered low value. Instead of the CDF, the government could have taken that money and put it into the normal health care system, where it would have benefited more patients (because of how the United Kingdom prioritizes care). For this reason, critics pounced. They wrote that the CDF "undermines the entire concept of a rational and evidence-based approach to the allocation of finite health-care resources" and, my favorite, the CDF is "already intellectually bankrupt."[4]

Throughout its tenure, the UK CDF was plagued with challenges. In 2016, a budget shortfall resulted in the fund cutting 45 drugs from the list of covered drugs. The list of cut medications was interesting. Thirty-eight percent improved survival, which was a higher percentage than the 30% of new FDA drug approvals that improved survival. In other words, the United Kingdom was cutting drugs that were better than the average drug coming to market in the United States. The fact that they were (1) not paid for by the traditional UK mechanism (aka not cost effective) and (2) ultimately cut from the CDF slush fund is just further evidence that the ability of nations, even large and wealthy ones like the United Kingdom, to negotiate cancer drug prices is limited.

I cannot resist recounting some of my favorite quotes about the

CDF. In 2014, the *Financial Times* wrote that the CDF is a "populist gesture that gives the impression of benefiting patients, but in fact rewards poor quality drugs while benefiting a handful of pharmaceutical companies at the expense of the taxpayer and the full range of NHS patients."[5] And one more, "This mechanism for diverting taxpayers' money to enhance, to little or no purpose, the profits of Big Pharma might be more aptly named 'the Drug Company Fund.' "[6]

What the situation with the CDF reveals about the United States is worrying. It can be argued that the US health care system is nothing more than a very large cancer drug fund that does not negotiate and never says no. In other words, Americans pay exorbitant sums of money for the same drugs used in the United Kingdom—and then some. Consider just one example. In the United States, we pay for 16 doses of brentuximab vedotin (Adcetris, Seattle Genetics) after a bone marrow transplant for Hodgkin's lymphoma based on an improvement in PFS, despite the fact that it has no survival benefit. If you think back to the principles I outline in chapter 10, this intervention appears to be foolish, as it extends the duration of therapy without a survival benefit. It adds cost and toxicity but has never shown survival gain. Here, the drug costs roughly $250,000, and we don't bat an eyelash. Meanwhile, the United Kingdom struggles to pay for the same brentuximab when used as a salvage agent, a setting where the cost is far lower and potential benefit larger.

The big lesson of the UK drug fund is that the cost of a medication is always paid by someone, and it means not paying for other things that would provide more value. In the United States, every dollar spent by the federal government on marginal cancer drugs is money we don't spend on cost-effective health care—like better care for people with obesity, high blood pressure, and those who are pregnant or have just had a baby. Many of these interventions would, dollar for dollar, be a far better use of our money. Even if cancer patients don't have a large copay, the horrendous price of cancer care makes all our premiums higher and diverts societal money that could otherwise be spent more wisely.

You might be thinking, "But what if I had terminal cancer?" It would be little comfort to know that, by you not getting a drug, it means some other person you have never met can be treated with blood pressure control. I agree and have a few thoughts on this. One, if the United States stopped paying any sum of money for poorly effective cancer drugs, companies would not develop these drugs. Rather, they may retool their entire R&D. They would likely pursue fewer drugs, and these drugs would have greater benefit and meet societal standards for cost-effectiveness. Thus, the situation where an individual patient feels cheated will diminish over time. Second, companies can alter the value of a medication at any time by lowering the price. Patients would directly pressure companies to do this. Currently, the fragmented system keeps many of us indifferent to drug prices. The easiest way to make a drug cost-effective is to lower the price. Third, in our lives, we all enter not knowing what will happen to us. Far more of us will have high blood pressure than die of cancer. The purpose of public policy is to maximize the welfare for the greatest number, without encroaching on individual freedoms. Policies that use societal money to pay for drugs with the biggest bang for the buck do just this. There will always be a place for individuals to use their own dollars as they best see fit, but we cannot fault a society that prioritizes payment for maternal care for 10,000 women, adding thousands of life-years to the world, over a pill that extends one person's life by one day. That society is not cruel, but just.

Clinical Trials in Low- and Middle-Income Countries

As I will discuss more in chapters 13 and 14, many companies conduct trials in places where they can use a control treatment that is not up to US standards or have post therapy care that is not up to US standards. In other words, they test a new drug against a drug known to be inferior to best practice or against a placebo. Moreover, after the trial, both groups often receive care far beneath the best US practice. In these cases, we are left uncertain as to whether that trial informs cancer care in the United States. This would be fine if the trial was intended to help the patients in the nation where the trial was conducted, but these trials are often registration studies meant to secure FDA approval. The FDA is essentially given cancer trial data that do not show how the drug would work in the United States. (Side note: the purpose of the FDA is to ensure safe and effective drugs in . . . you guessed it . . . the United States.)

However, to truly understand the debate around how to conduct trials globally, we must first draw some distinctions. Some global trials are like the aforementioned cancer drug trials—really meant for regulatory approval in the United States and Europe, and they should be subject to certain considerations. Other global trials are meant to inform the practice of locals living in those nations. In the 1990s, several clinical trials conducted in Africa, of the latter type, set off a longstanding debate that now has particular relevance for cancer clinical trials conducted globally.

In the 1990s, we knew that full doses of HIV medication could reduce the rate at which HIV-positive mothers transmitted the virus to their offspring, but the reality was that these drugs remained unaffordable in many parts of the world, including Africa. Several trials, partly funded by the US National Institutes of Health and Centers for Disease Control, tested whether shorter treatment courses or lower doses of the HIV medication could still lower the rate of transmission. To do this, they tested these drugs against placebo, which ignited a firestorm.

All trials are designed to answer a question. If you test a full dose of HIV medication against a half dose, you can ask whether half the total dose is non-inferior. But, if you want to know whether a half dose is better than doing nothing, you have to test the half dose against placebo. Prior to the controversial studies in Africa, the reality was that nearly no one in Africa was getting the full dose of the HIV medication. Thus, investigators of these studies tested the second question. Many felt that this design was unethical, but it alone was capable of asking the question that faced local populations. Since this book is about cancer, I will leave the debate there (it was unresolved) and pick it up over a decade later when it reemerged with a cancer study.

A Trial of Cervical Cancer Screening

In 2014 a randomized trial was published that showed that, in a Mumbai slum, visual inspection of the cervix could lower deaths from cervical cancer. The control arm of the study was no screening, which was actually the state of living in that slum at the time of the study. Because the control arm did not get Pap smears, many were outraged.[7]

The world is not fair. It is neither fair nor just that millions of people live in nations without access to basic health care, yet this is the reality of 2018. Currently, in nearly all of India, women do not have access to the Papanicolaou test (or Pap smear). Why? Because it is too expensive. For this reason, many women there go unscreened for cervical cancer, and the death rate from cervical cancer in India is large. In fact, 72,000 women, or 26% of all women globally who die of cervical cancer, die in India.[8]

With that backdrop, researchers from Tata Memorial Centre in Mumbai, India, conducted a randomized trial where low-cost, low-skilled community health workers were trained and deployed into Indian slums.[9] There the workers looked at a woman's cervix with their own eyes after applying a vinegar solution (acetic acid). Early cancerous and precancerous lesions have a characteristic appearance. If any were seen, the community health workers treated these with local therapies. The trial showed that this intervention, which was affordable and scalable, could lower cervical cancer death. Some estimated that the intervention could save 22,000 lives a year.[10] Again, critics asked why the control arm of women received nothing.

Thus far in this book, I hope I have convinced you that historically controlled or nonrandomized trials would be unable to answer this question. Anything short of a randomized trial could be affected by bias and lead to misleading conclusions, and given that we need a randomized trial, the choice was either: test the visual inspection of the cervix with acetic acid (VIA) against the Pap smear or test it against doing nothing. If you ran the first study, as some wish, you might get really lucky to find the VIA is non-inferior (with a proper margin; see chapter 11) or really lucky to find that it is even better than the Pap smear! But, this is unlikely to be the case. VIA is probably worse than the Pap smear, but is it better than doing nothing—the de facto standard? The answer to that question cannot be known unless you test the intervention against doing nothing. That's what the researchers did.

In 2014, Sham Mailankody, Hemanth Kumar, and I argued in the *Journal of Global Oncology* that there is a generalizable principle here.[7] You can test an intervention against doing nothing or placebo in a low- or middle-income country if doing nothing is the current standard of care and, if positive, the intervention you are testing could be scaled up. In other words, if the trial results could positively impact the population, then it can be ethically conducted in resource-poor countries. If you go to the Mumbai slum and test a brand new $20,000 genetic test for cervical cancer, what good will that be? Women there cannot afford a Pap smear, and they certainly will not be able to afford the new test. Nevertheless, if you test something that is cheap and scalable, then you are on to something. A positive trial could really make the world a better place. Unfortunately, many new cancer drug trials don't meet the second part of our principle.

Modern Cancer Drug Trials

Trastuzumab is a monoclonal antibody directed against HER2, which is a target for some women with breast cancer. In 2001, a randomized trial showed that adding trastuzumab to chemotherapy improved survival by five months (from 20 months to 25 months).[11] By 2005, there was accumulating evidence that continuing trastuzumab after progression may continue to exert benefit.[17] A year later, from 2006 to 2009, over 400 women in China with HER2-positive breast cancer were randomized to chemotherapy with or without lapatinib, a new HER2 drug. These patients did not get trastuzumab.

This might be okay if the price was far lower for lapatinib than trastuzumab, but it wasn't. In fact, based on 2014 prices listed in Redbook—a database of average wholesale pharmacy prices—one year of treatment costs $66,000 for trastuzumab and $67,000 for lapatinib.

What sense does this make? We already know an HER2-positive

drug improves survival, and that drug is trastuzumab. If you have over $60,000 a year and have HER2-positive breast cancer, that is the drug you should get. What good would it do to prove lapatinib does the same thing at a cost of a thousand dollars more? Notably, this trial could not be performed elsewhere, as doctors would not be comfortable withholding trastuzumab from patients assigned to the control arm. Instead, this trial should have compared lapatinib to trastuzumab to prove added benefit. Lapatinib isn't the only culprit. Another example of a questionable trial design is the case of afatinib.

Afatinib (Boehringer Ingelheim, Germany) is a targeted inhibitor of EGFR. By the time it came to market, we already had two other EGFR inhibitors—erlotinib and gefitinib. In August of 2009, a randomized trial was published showing gefitinib was superior* to chemotherapy for patients with activating mutations of EGFR.[13] That same month, a randomized trial of afatinib began testing essentially the exact same question in a Chinese population: "Is afatinib better than chemotherapy?"[14] It was one of two similar trials.[15]

What sense do these trials make? If anything, afatinib should be tested against gefitinib because gefitinib had just been shown to be superior to chemotherapy. The afatinib investigators may protest that they had already planned their trial before the results of the other study were published. Okay, sure, but they should change their plans because new information came out. You can't be so wedded to your plans when those plans involve subjecting half of your patients to a treatment already known to be inferior to chemotherapy.

On the other hand, you might argue that gefitinib is costly and essentially out of reach for most people in China. There is a desperate need to find a cheaper option. Thus, just like the VIA trial in India, we are testing afatinib. However, this argument falls short because afatinib costs $79,000 per year, while gefitinib costs $25,000 per year. Gefitinib is a bargain in comparison to afatinib.

* This whole discussion concerns progression-free and not overall survival, but that doesn't change anything, as all studies pursued the same goal. Nevertheless, if you want to argue that we didn't know if there was an overall survival benefit of gefitinib, the afatinib trial wasn't designed to answer that, either. You cannot have it both ways.

So why did researchers run this trial in low- and middle-income* countries? Probably because it would be very difficult to run this trial in the United States and Western Europe, where we had already started using erlotinib and gefitinib. No self-respecting physicians in the United States would allow their patients to be randomized to chemotherapy. The only way to run such a study is to go somewhere where patients don't have access to the already approved EGFR drugs.

Both afatinib and lapatinib fail the second part of our ethics test. It is not okay to test a new drug against a substandard comparator or an older drug that is not currently used. I believe it is exploitative to conduct trials in low- and middle-income countries just to get more next-in-class drugs on the US market. There has to be a better way.

Which Trials Should Be Conducted in Low- and Middle-Income Countries?

I want to end part III (on global oncology) with some thoughts about amazing research that can occur in low- and middle-income countries, which have potential to perform good RCTs that test important hypotheses. These aren't trials that exploit the country but ones that ask a question relevant to the health care and practices of the country, and perhaps even the globe. Here are some selected trials that show what is possible.

Removing the Primary Tumor in Cancer That Has Spread

In cancer medicine, if a solid tumor has already spread to distant sites, there is only one reason to give local treatment to the primary, or starting, site. If the primary site is causing symptoms, and by treating it we

* In this chapter, I use the phrase *low- and middle-income country* (LMIC)—not *developing country* or a prior term that was in vogue (e.g., *third world country*). At the time I wrote this book, LMIC was considered the most appropriate and least pejorative term to use. However, future readers may see this as pejorative, just as *third world* is considered today. Let me be clear. I have nothing against these fine nations. They do their best with a world that is economically unfair, and I hope future readers forgive my terminology if the vernacular shifts again.

can ameliorate those symptoms, then we would give local treatment. If the primary tumor is not causing symptoms,* then treating it is generally considered a fool's errand. It is analogous to closing the barn door after the horse has bolted.

There is one exception. In kidney cancer, it was long hypothesized that the primary tumor fostered the growth of distant sites. Of course, this was just a hypothesis that needed to be tested. In a rigorous randomized trial to determine whether to remove the kidney or not, a survival advantage was shown with the removal of the affected kidney, which is why we perform this intervention in metastatic kidney cancer today.[16] Yet, this trial was done prior to the advent of novel medications to treat kidney cancer. When a modern version was reattempted comparing surgery to new drugs, there no longer was a benefit.[17] There are two lessons here. First, the one example I had of removing a primary tumor in metastatic disease to improve survival did not stand the test of time (its efficacy changed as I was writing the book), and second, we must reassess our beliefs as medical practice changes. The same intervention that worked in 1980 may no longer be effective in the landscape of 2020, or vice versa.

When it comes to breast cancer, observational studies have repeatedly tried to address the question of whether removing the primary tumor in metastatic disease was beneficial. Here is just a quick summary.

In 2002, an observational study of the National Cancer Database found that removing the primary breast cancer after the tumor had spread dramatically improved survival, with a hazard ratio of 0.61.[18] If true, this would be about twice the benefit of that seen in 2001 with trastuzumab, which is a good drug in the metastatic setting.[11] What I am trying to say is that the benefit here seems too good to be true. It seems unlikely that removing a portion of cancer is better for a person than a highly effective systemic drug.

In 2006, another two observational papers came forward to show that removing the primary breast tumor, even after the cancer had

---

* This could be where symptoms are pending. As you can imagine, this is a very gray zone.

spread, could improve survival.[19,20] In 2007, two more observational papers were added to the pile[21,22] and two more in 2008.[23,24]

Now, 2012 was a momentous year. For years, I had been saying that a meta-analysis is like an automatic fruit juicer. The juice only tastes as good as what you put in the juicer, and people have been putting a lot of rotting fruit in the juicer. In that vein, a meta-analysis of these (weak) observational studies showed that removing the primary cancer in patients with metastatic breast cancer saved lives. The hazard ratio was 0.69, and the p-value had lots of zeros in it![25]

What was wrong with all these studies? (The real question is what is wrong with the researchers who believe these studies are actually providing useful information?) There is something different about the people on whom surgery was performed versus those on whom it was not performed. It might be the aggressiveness of their doctor, but it could also be that they were fit, willing, and motivated to do this unproven thing. Patients who didn't look well enough in the eyes of the physician were probably selected out. This phenomenon is called *confounding by indication*. In this case, the people who got the procedure done were healthier than those who didn't get it. If the patients who did not get the surgery were as healthy as those who did get the surgery, then they would have likely had the procedure too! In other words, being healthy led to the procedure, which would make it falsely look like the procedure resulted in better survival.

The only way to answer whether an invasive or toxic cancer therapy improves survival is through a randomized trial, and though several are ongoing for surgery in metastatic breast cancer, only one has been completed and published. That study comes from the Tata Medical Centre in Mumbai, India, which has consistently shown just how excellent research can be from a low- and middle-income country.

Between 2005 and 2013, researchers at Tata randomized more than 700 patients with metastatic cancer to either removal of the breast and axillary nodes plus chemotherapy or chemotherapy alone. A picture is worth a thousand words, and figure 12.1 shows the survival curve of the two groups. Both groups start with everyone alive, with patients passing away over time.[26]

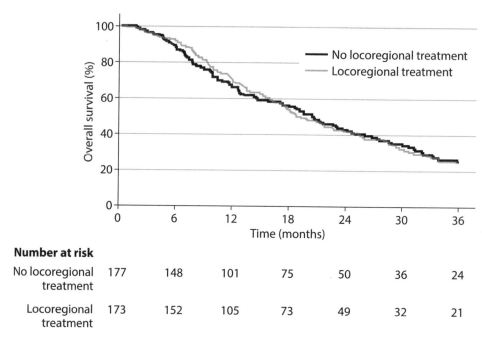

Number at risk

No locoregional treatment	177	148	101	75	50	36	24
Locoregional treatment	173	152	105	73	49	32	21

Figure 12.1. Kaplan-Meier plot of overall survival. Comparing locoregional treatment versus no treatment of the primary tumor in metastatic breast cancer. Used with permission by the *Lancet Oncology.*

There is absolutely no difference between the two groups, suggesting that many of the prior observational studies and that garbage in garbage out (GIGO) meta-analysis were all off the mark. While leading cancer centers around the globe wasted their time churning out retrospective studies, the folks at Tata ran the correct trial that was capable of answering the question of the effectiveness of locoregional treatment.

Comparing Two Doses of Chemotherapy

The second study I want to highlight also comes from Tata. There have been two ways to give cisplatin with radiation in the curative treatment of head and neck cancer. The first way was to give it at a high dose every three weeks. The newer way is to give it at a lower dose every week. A lot of doctors switched to the lower dose every week because they believed it was easier for patients, but they didn't know which was more effective. The folks at Tata ran the randomized trial comparing the two and found some suggestion that every three weeks was superior.[27] It might sound trivial, but as we learned (with gemtuzumab ozogamicin in chapter 2), the right drug at the wrong dose can harm patients.

Conclusion

The take-home lesson is that low- and middle-income countries can perform important research that benefits citizens both of those nations and around the world. Although they are increasingly seduced by high-tech therapies with marginal (if any) gains and large price tags, they would be best served by focusing on what truly matters. Low- and middle-income nations can test the necessity of surgeries, commonly used medications, variations in dose, and variations in schedule (how often a drug is administered). You don't need to have all the fancy new drugs to answer fundamental questions about cancer medicine. You just need to be organized and diligent, and embrace the power of randomization. You must question dogma without data. I expect more great work to come from these nations in the years to come, and I end here with a table of other great trials from Tata (table 12.1).

Table 12.1. Selected list of cancer trials from Tata Memorial Centre, Mumbai, India

Title	Authors	Description
Elective versus Therapeutic Neck Dissection in Node-Negative Oral Cancer[a]	Anil K. D'Cruz, MS, DNB, Richa Vaish, MS, Neeti Kapre, MS, DNB, Mitali Dandekar, MS, DNB, Sudeep Gupta, MD, DM, Rohini Hawaldar, BSc, DCM, Jai Prakash Agarwal, MD, Gouri Pantvaidya, MS, DNB, Devendra Chaukar, MS, DNB, Anuja Deshmukh, MS, DLO, DORL, Shubhada Kane, MD, Supreeta Arya, MD, DNB, DMRD, et al., for the Head and Neck Disease Management Group	Prospective, randomized, controlled trial of 596 patients with early-stage, clinically node-negative oral squamous-cell cancer comparing elective neck dissection to therapeutic neck dissection. After three years, elective node dissection resulted in an improved rate of overall survival (80.0%; 95% confidence interval [CL], 74.1 to 85.8) compared with therapeutic dissection (95% CI, 0.45 to 0.92; $p = 0.01$).
Effect of VIA Screening by Primary Health Workers: Randomized Controlled Study in Mumbai, India[b]	Surendra S. Shastri, Indraneel Mittra, Gauravi A. Mishra, Subhadra Gupta, Rajesh Dikshit, Shalini Singh, Rajendra A. Badwe	Cluster-randomized controlled study examining visual inspection of the cervix after application of 4% acetic acid (VIA), as an alternative to a Pap smear–based national screening program. This trial found that VIA screening by primary health workers could prevent 22,000 cervical cancer deaths in India and 72,600 deaths in resource-poor countries annually.

[a]D'Cruz AK, Vaish R, Kapre N, et al. Elective versus therapeutic neck dissection in node-negative oral cancer. *New England Journal of Medicine.* 2015;373(6):521–529.
[b]Shastri SS, Mittra I, Mishra GA, et al. Effect of VIA screening by primary health workers: randomized controlled study in Mumbai, India. *JNCI: Journal of the National Cancer Institute.* 2014;106(3):dju009–dju009.

PART IV **SOLUTIONS**

THIRTEEN

How Should Cancer Drug Development Proceed?

Randomize the first patient.

THOMAS CHALMERS

OVER THE preceding chapters, we have seen that the incentives for cancer drug development engender practices that are not consistent with either their stated goal or, more importantly, the patients' best interests. We have seen that drug developers may trade the speed a surrogate provides for the size of the market share. Specifically, in chapter 2, I discussed two HER2-directed drugs; one showed a survival benefit in the second line of therapy, and the other showed a PFS benefit in the front line. Both trials took similar time to complete, but one reaped a larger market share. Instead of a surrogate bringing a drug to market faster for people with relapsed tumors, companies may use the surrogate in the untreated (front-line) cancer to get a bigger market share.

We have also seen that the profits at stake, billions and billions of dollars, are disconnected from the benefit the drugs provide. These profits encourage companies to conduct larger and larger studies, hoping to squeeze out a statistically significant p-value of 0.04999 or less. As long as you show a statistically significant improvement in survival, typically defined as a p-value less than 0.05, it doesn't matter how long or short the actual benefit is, whether it is clinically meaningful or not. That's why erlotinib in pancreatic cancer is FDA approved with a 10-day median survival benefit. The massive profit for marginal drugs incentivizes companies to move forward with drugs without much potential benefit.

Finally, we have seen that, likely out of a desire to use the accelerated approval pathway, nearly any cancer condition has been called an "unmet medical need." It doesn't matter if that cancer already has dozens of treatment options, has a favorable prognosis, and is fairly common.

Here, I will describe the framework for an alternative system. With a few minor tweaks, we can encourage more rational drug development that is in the best interest of people with cancer. This system would, in my opinion, lead to good drugs coming to market faster and bad drugs rejected sooner, and it may lead companies to retool their entire R&D apparatus to chase good drugs, not merely marginal drugs that can get approval. Of course, I want to begin with a disclaimer that, as with any proposal, I ask that my ideas be tested as they are implemented and not immediately accepted simply because they make sense. Good policy has to be empirically validated, not just plausible.

How Bad Is the Current System?

A seminal moment in the life of a cancer drug occurs when it is tested in a phase 1, first-in-human trial. Prior to this moment, the data supporting drugs come from animal studies, petri dishes full of cancer cells, and other laboratory experiments. Although one would wish these preclinical studies had tremendous ability to predict which drugs would succeed, the truth is far from this. That is why in chapter 5, I faulted the media for calling drugs only given to mice "miracles" and "game changers." The chance that drugs with promising animal trials will succeed in humans is low.

The stated purpose of phase 1 trials is to establish the ideal dose for subsequent testing. But, truth be told, we are looking for more than just that. Ideally, you would see some evidence of activity, such as tumor response, in these studies. Maybe just a couple patients have their cancer shrink. If no cancer patient has a response, a phase 1 could still be successful, that is, the dose for future studies found, but many oncologists won't be too happy with this outcome.

Drugs without overt toxicity move forward to phase 2, which seeks to establish evidence of drug activity. These are often nonrandomized, and the primary endpoint is to show that the response rate is greater than some prespecified threshold.[1] Some writers have argued that more of these trials should be randomized and that randomization should be implemented even earlier.[2] This is a sound proposal.

Phase 3 trials are the final (preapproval) step of drug testing and typically use a randomized design to show a new therapy is better than current practice. There is no consensus on what needs to be shown in a phase 2 trial in order to advance to phase 3. There isn't even consensus on whether you need a proper phase 2 to move on to a phase 3 trial. Throughout this book, I have tried to suggest that the current incentive structure actually encourages drug companies to be less selective in advancing to phase 3 trials. The payoff for a phase 3 success is so great, even long odds are worth taking.

In 2017, some colleagues and I performed a thought experiment to illustrate just how bad things had gotten.[3] But first, we need to clarify a few things. In our study, which looked at the cost of R&D to bring a new cancer drug to market (discussed in chapters 1 and 4 of this book), we found that in just four years on the market, the median revenue earned by a cancer drug was $1.65 billion. On average, drugs have 14 years on the market, and revenue only gets bigger with more time on the market. In fact, investigators from the World Health Organization found that the average cancer drug earns over 10 billion dollars in revenue, an average during the 14 years of exclusivity it enjoys in the United States.[4] That's a lot of money. But, running trials costs a lot of money too. It turns out that the cost to run a randomized trial in oncology has been pegged at $22 million.[5]

So, consider a wild idea—an implausible, worst-case scenario. Imagine I worked at a pharmaceutical company. Imagine I have access to large libraries of chemical compounds. Imagine that the truth about most of these drugs is that, at a low dose, they are inert. They neither help nor harm. What if I just picked 100 of these compounds and tested them each in large phase 3 randomized trials?

Such a proposal would sound insane. After all, these drugs are inert.

They have no real chance of helping cancer patients. Moreover, the cost to test 100 drugs would be astronomical— $2.2 billion in fact, if you assumed it costs $22 million per randomized trial, as I just told you. And for what? What would you have to gain by this seemingly ridiculous idea?

Quite a lot, in fact. If you test 100 inert compounds in randomized trials and used a one-tailed p-value of 0.05 as the bar for significance, five trials will have significant results, on average, by chance alone. This number may even be higher if you add in the bias that comes from randomized trials. That means your $2.2 billion outlay would get you five drug approvals. And given that the WHO investigators point out the average drug earns $10 billion in revenue, you might make $50 billion from these five drugs. This is particularly true if the FDA has no minimum survival benefit requirement—not to worry, it doesn't—and is willing to approve drugs based on one trial—also, in luck, that's the way it is.

So, consider the question: at what point does it become financially beneficial to test completely inert substances? If conducting one trial can get an approval, if it doesn't matter what the magnitude of benefit is, and if it doesn't matter what other trials show (think sunitinib, in chapter 10), then becomes silly not to test useless compounds. In this case, spending 2.2 billion on 100 chemicals with no promise would get five approvals by false positive alone. That would leave you with $47.8 billion in your pocket (5 × $10 billion (revenue post approval) – $2.2 billion (cost to run trials).* In other words, the current incentives around drug approval are so perverted that a company could get rich from testing totally useless things.

Of course, I do not believe that the current drug approval process is as bad as this scenario, but I worry that *it is not a whole lot better*. Consider the EVOLVE-1 study.[6] EVOLVE-1 randomized 546 patients with liver cancer that had progressed on the standard therapy to either everolimus or placebo. The trial was negative and cost the company a

* If you prefer a two-tailed p-value, the calculation would be $25 billion – $2.2 billion, or $22.8 billion in your pocket.

great deal. And yet, in the EVOLVE-1 paper, the authors admit that a large randomized trial was launched solely on the results of laboratory studies and a small phase 1 / phase 2 trial, showing that the drug might work. In other words, there wasn't a lot of clinical information that the company had before it pulled the trigger on a large, costly phase 3 trial. One might imagine a more prudent thing would be for researchers to do a small, randomized phase 2 trial first. So why didn't they?

At the time of this writing, there are at least 10 published phase 3 trials in metastatic liver cancer,[7] and, with the exception of sorafenib, none improved outcomes in the front line. (Remember brivanib from chapter 11 and that sorafenib itself did not look that good in the real world in chapter 1.) The only other positive trials we have in liver cancer are in the second-line setting. Lenvatinib was a notable non-inferiority trial (chapter 11). Many of the drugs tested have been very similar to sorafenib. Before sorafenib, several cytotoxic drugs had failed to generate high responses in this setting. Put another way, it is clear that hepatocellular cancer (HCC) is a tough cancer, and most of our drugs fall short. At the same time, you see a drug industry testing compounds with very little phase 3 rationale—as in the case of everolimus. That doesn't make a lot of sense unless the reward for a fluke positive result was so great that it would justify a dozen or more failed trials.

Bishal Gyawali and Alfredo Addeo surveyed one year of negative phase 3 randomized controlled trials[8] in the top cancer journals. They found 12 negative randomized trials of novel cancer drugs. Of these 12, they found one trial (8.3%) conducted without a phase 2 study, three (25%) conducted despite negative phase 2 studies, five (42%) conducted based on inconclusive phase 2 studies, and only three (25%) conducted based on positive phase 2 studies. As long as the bar for approval is one single positive phase 3 trial and the financial reward for an approval is billions of dollars, we will continue to see large clinical trial agendas of dubious rationale.

Finally, it is worth commenting about the size of a clinical trial. The right clinical trial is sized to rule in a meaningful clinical benefit. Adrian Sacher and colleagues noted that over time in oncology, the median sample size has been increasing in phase 3 trials. That results in added cost and increased precision, but it also permits the detection of small, statistically significant benefits of dubious clinical value. They found a decreasing magnitude of benefit was considered "positive" over time in lung cancer.[9] When you couple this with the observation in chapter 2 by Kay and colleagues of the shifting endpoints in oncology, you may conclude that our lofty prices and low regulatory standards are incentivizing the industry to develop marginal drugs—drugs tested in trials that can detect the tiniest difference in progression-free survival.

Along these lines, Del Paggio and colleagues[10] looked at the power calculation in scientific papers to ask how many randomized trials assess clinically meaningful benefits. They found that just 31% (70/226) of trials met this bar, while most test benefits are not clinically meaningful (aka smaller, marginal benefits). Moreover, this is an optimistic estimate, as the authors use the point estimate of the effect and not the lower bound of the confidence interval to make their assessment. If you didn't understand that last sentence, move on, it isn't critical. The bottom line is simple. Our current regulatory system is the parent that spoils the child. We buy our sons and daughters a BMW or Ferrari for a D+ report card and then wonder why they don't work harder for A's?

Which Drugs Should Be Pursued?

One more piece of evidence to show that we test drugs in phase 3 trials with a hair trigger is the continual pursuit of drugs without single agent activity. Single agent activity means that a new drug, by itself, is capable of some degree of tumor shrinkage (some response) in patients with the type of cancer in which you are pursuing the drug. Over the years, I had felt that any drug worth its salt has single agent activity. In 2016, Bishal Gyawali and I put it to the test.[11]

We identified all drugs approved by the FDA in the prior 10 years that came to market solely in combination with other drugs with single agent activity and not by themselves. This is a methodological way to tease out the drugs that lack single agent activity that were nevertheless pursued and successfully approved. Most of these drugs had response rates of less than 10%. Keep in mind that response rates from sugar pills have been known to creep as high as 7%, due to the issues I explored in chapters 2 and 3.[12] In short, these drugs are ones that don't do much in and of themselves, but companies nevertheless successfully brought them to market, always in combination with already approved drugs.

We looked at this list (table 13.1) and noted that the median improvement in overall survival was 1.6 months. The median improvement in PFS was 2.3 months. The single biggest survival advantage was with bevacizumab (Avastin, Roche), but as I discussed in chapter 9, if you look at the portfolio of bevacizumab trials, this stands out as an outlier, so take it with a grain of salt. These were considered the success stories. Can you imagine how the drugs without single agent activity performed that didn't make it to approval?

For this reason, I would argue that drugs without single agent activity should generally not be pursued, unless there is some extraordinary evidence of synergy,* and there usually is not. By abandoning drugs that lack single agent activity, we will save tremendous amounts of money. We will miss out on a handful of ineffective drugs and a few extremely marginal ones. The capital we free can instead be used to pursue more meaningful targets.

This would be my first principle of cancer drug development. Evidence of drug activity is not proof that a drug benefits patients, but it is a reasonable, general prerequisite for moving forward to randomized trials. All of the truly transformational drugs in oncology have single agent activity in the metastatic setting. If the incentives around drugs were different, we might see companies make the decision to advance drugs only with sound rationale to randomized trial.

Which Patients Should Come First in Phase 3 Trials?

Cancer drugs should first be tested in randomized trials of severe, advanced disease states, unless there is a strong reason why they should

---

* If you want to learn more about additive cancer drug benefit and synergy, you would do well to read this article: Palmer AC, Sorger PK. Combination cancer therapy can confer benefit via patient-to-patient variability without drug additivity or synergy. Cell.171(7):1678–1691,e1613.

Table 13.1. Approvals of drugs with limited evidence of single agent activity as combination therapies

Year of FDA approval	Drug	Approved indication (advanced-stage)	Combination partner(s)	Approval end point	Improvement in OS (median)	Improvement in PFS/TTP (median)	PMID
Drugs targeting the VEGF-signaling pathway							
2015	Ramucirumab	Colorectal cancer	FOLFIRI	OS	1.6 months	1.2 months	25877855
2014	Ramucirumab	NSCLC	Docetaxel	OS	1.4 months	1.5 months	24933332
2014	Bevacizumab	Ovarian, fallopian tube, or peritoneal cancer	Paclitaxel, Doxil, or topotecan	PFS	NS	3.3 months	24637997
2014	Bevacizumab	Cervical cancer	Paclitaxel + cisplatin or topotecan	OS	3.7 months	2.3 months	24552320
2013	Bevacizumab	Colorectal cancer	FOLFOX or FOLFIRI	OS	1.4 months	1.6 months	23168366
2012	Ziv-aflibercept	Colorectal cancer	FOLFIRI	OS	1.4 months	2.2 months	22949147
2009	Bevacizumab	Renal-cell cancer	IFN-α	PFS	NS	4.8 months	18156031
Drugs used to treat breast cancer							
2016	Palbociclib	HR+HER2– breast cancer	Fulvestrant	PFS	NR	4.9 months	26947331
2012	Everolimus	HR+HER2– breast cancer	Exemestane	PFS	NS	4.1 months	22149876, 25231953
2010	Lapatinib	HR+ HER2+ breast cancer	Letrozole	PFS	NS	5.2 months	19786658
2007	Lapatinib	HER2+ breast cancer	Capecitabine	TTP	NS	1.9 months	18188694

Drugs used to treat multiple myeloma

Year	Drug	Indication	Endpoint			PMID
2015	Elotuzumab	Multiple myeloma	PFS and ORR	NR	4.5 months	26035255
2015	Panobinostat	Multiple myeloma	PFS	NS (immature)	3.8 months	25242045
2007	Liposomal doxorubicin	Multiple myeloma	TTP	NS	2.8 months	17679727
Drugs used to treat pancreatic cancer						
2015	Liposomal irinotecan	Pancreatic cancer	OS	1.9 months	1.6 months	26615328
2013	Nab-paclitaxel	Pancreatic cancer	OS	1.8 months	1.8 months	24131140
Other drugs						
2015	Necitumumab	NSCLC	OS	1.6 months	0.2 months	26045340
2010	Trastuzumab	Gastric or gastroesophageal junction cancer	OS	2.7 months	1.2 months	20728210

Note: We examined all drugs that received FDA approval over the past decade[a] and identified the drugs approved only in combinations, then excluded those that have also been approved as single agents for the same disease. Efficacy data comes from the FDA drug label or published study of the pivotal trial (PMID provided).

5-FU, 5-fluorouracil; Doxil, pegylated liposomal doxorubicin; FOLFIRI, 5-FU, folinic acid and irinotecan; FOLFOX, 5-FU, folinic acid and oxaliplatin; HR, hormone receptor; NR, not reported; NS, not significant; NSCLC, non-small-cell lung cancer; ORR, objective response rate; OS, overall survival; PFS, progression-free survival; PMID, PubMed identification number; TTP, time to tumor progression; VEGF, vascular endothelial growth factor.

[a]US FDA. Hematology/oncology (cancer) approvals & safety notifications. In US H, ed. [Online]: US Food & Drug Administration, 2017.

be tested elsewhere, which is usually not the case.[13] This is true for a few reasons. First, we want to measure endpoints that matter to patients, such as overall survival or quality of life. Second, trials to assess survival will be completed more rapidly in settings where the event occurs more rapidly. In other words, the fastest you can show a drug improves survival is in a group of people who are facing a life-threatening problem. And third, we won't miss winners. As noted in chapter 10, all drugs that work in the adjuvant setting also have activity in the metastatic setting, while the reverse is not true. Many drugs that work in the metastatic setting fail in the adjuvant setting. Fourth, patients in the last line have typically exhausted other proven treatment options and are most in need of novel treatment options, and perhaps are most willing to tolerate the risk of trials. The fifth reason is that this method provides a clear and logical way to advance drugs earlier in the treatment of disease (more to come on that).

As an aside, I should clarify that trials that assess survival produce results faster in more lethal situations. This is generally the last-line setting but not always the last line. If a researcher uses very restrictive inclusion criteria, it is possible to select patients in later lines with nearly the same survival as those with untreated cancer. For instance, survival in the control arms of sorafenib versus best supportive care (front-line hepatocellular cancer) and regorafenib versus best supportive care (second-line hepatocellular cancer) are nearly identical, largely driven by patient selection. The conventional teaching that patients with relapsed cancer are sicker than those with newly diagnosed cancer doesn't take into account the selection bias that happens. In my vision of drug development, we would have little to no selection bias, and thus ensure drugs are tested in patients reflective of the actual population of people with cancer (more to come in chapter 14).

If we agree that active drugs should first be tested in later lines of therapy, then let's also agree that these drugs be tested against the best available US standard of care—whether that be supportive care, a palliative cytotoxic supported by phase 2 trial, or a targeted drug.

Finally, let me reiterate that the primary endpoint of these trials must be overall survival. Cancer is highly lethal, and we need drugs to improve survival. Quality of life must also be routinely measured, but if a drug improves quality of life alone, we still need adequate power to exclude a survival decrement. And, the truth is that highly effective cancer drugs usually improve both survival and quality of life.

The concern that routinely demanding proof of survival benefit would slow drugs reaching the market is unjustified because, as we have seen in chapter 2, using surrogates to speed this process may have the paradoxical effect of encouraging companies to move to the front line, trading speed for market share. Work I collaborated on, led by Emerson Chen,[14] found that the time savings associated with using surrogates is only 12%. Moreover, I have already stated that initial trials should be performed in the last line. Because these patients have limited survival, it would be neither difficult nor time consuming to show a survival benefit. Chen's work finds no time savings in this line. Finally, if the treatment truly works, it should be approved immediately.

The de facto endpoint of overall survival may be suspended in cases that are truly "unmet medical needs"—conditions that are actually dire and lethal with no options. Here, surrogates can be used for accelerated approval. Of course, it goes without saying that trials assessing overall survival should be completed postmarket. Finally, whether or not one or two trials is sufficient is a complex, empirical question that I will set aside for now. Remember that in other diseases, conducting two trials is the norm.

Finally, and we will discuss this more in the next chapter, one does not need to do much to the current system to encourage or nudge the industry to move to the model I suggest. If the FDA demanded that cancer drugs improve overall survival before coming to market and that control arms be fair and up to US standards, you would see the industry abide by my suggestions. It would be logical to conduct trials in last lines of therapy first—for the sake of speed and size.

How to Advance Drugs?

Now, what happens to a drug that succeeds in the last line of therapy? For drugs that come to market—that show improved outcomes in relapsed cancer—attempts should be made to move them to earlier lines of therapy. The burden that faces these drugs is to prove that earlier administration of the agent (for example, second-line rather than third-line multiple myeloma or front-line rather than second-line non-small-cell lung cancer) is superior to using the drug in the later line, as has already been validated.

Here, crossover must be mandatory. The salient question is whether early administration of this drug improves outcomes beyond administration upon progression. Moreover, if the trial is intended to guide US drug approval (it usually is), it cannot be conducted in countries with standard of care inferior to that of the United States, where patients do not have access to the drug in later lines for reasons discussed in chapter 12.

For drugs that succeed in improving overall survival in the front-line metastatic space, they should be tested, where appropriate, against current best therapy in the adjuvant space. This is the most logical way to maximize the use of drugs, while ensuring that all decisions are based on evidence and data, not hope and hype.

What Is the Best Dose? And in Whom?

Another part of the cancer drug research agenda must be to test variations in dosing and schedule. In other words, all patients get proven drugs, but we test whether starting at a lower dose and ramping up is superior to the approved dosing or whether a lower dose given weekly is superior to the approved every three-week dosing. In the current world, there is very little optimization of drug dosing that happens post-market, and what little there is of it is driven by biological thinking. A robust system would create a formalized way of exploring variations in dosing via randomized trial.

Finally, novel biomarkers can be explored. Is there a genetic signature that identifies patients who do not benefit? If so, the corollary must also be true: the signature identifies patients who have a *greater* benefit on average, as it excludes the ones for whom the drug does not work. A robust, federally funded trial agenda can answer these vital questions.

As we have seen, the industry has little incentive to develop a test that will only erode its market share.

How Should Trials Be Structured?

Given the problems I have described in preceding chapters, there are several solutions to strengthen the structure of cancer trials. First, trials should generally be randomized and have the primary endpoint of overall survival.[15] Adapting randomization based on interim outcomes or skewed ratios of randomization are suboptimal and may even be detrimental.[15] Second, patients should be enrolled as if they would receive the drug in the real world, without restriction on age, comorbidities, or fitness. Unless there is a strong biological reason to exclude some medical problem, which there rarely is,[16] patients should be put on the study. Ideally, some sort of computerized system should be in place nationally so that patients can be enrolled on trials at any site in the country, whether or not they live close to an anointed cancer center.

The control arm should receive the best available drugs. For instance, ibrutinib should not be tested against single agent chlorambucil (more to come on this topic in the next chapter). The dose of the control-arm medication should be fair. There should be no rules against concomitant medications that would otherwise be used in standard practice. For instance, you can't restrict the antinausea medication a doctor might use.

If you want to measure response or progression (even if it is not your primary endpoint) the trial must be double-blinded—with neither patients nor doctors aware of assignment. The quality of blinding should be assessed. It should not be open label, which is a common design feature that may distort outcomes. For instance, investigators who know that a patient is getting a control-arm drug may be more likely to declare progression of the disease, which would hasten the end of the trial, in order to administer alternative therapy believed to be more effective.

The backbone, or control-arm, drugs have to be the ones that are actually used, and if you want to inform US practice, use the backbone that is already used in the United States. For instance, the US standard of care for multiple myeloma is bortezomib (Velcade) plus lenalidomide (Revlimid) and dexamethasone (VRd) not bortezomib plus melphalan and prednisone (VMP). There are many other commonsense design elements that ensure a fair fight. Who designs these trials is the key to make them all happen.

How Should the Trial Be Powered?

How the trial should be powered is a major consideration. A trial's power essentially means what difference between the two arms is capable of being detected as significant. A trial should be powered to assess a meaningful benefit. Currently, trials are overpowered to find statistically significant but clinically meaningless benefits. Cancer trials should be powered to find benefits at least as big as those proposed by the American Society of Clinical Oncology (ASCO) and European Society for Medical Oncology (ESMO) guidelines. These are minimum improvements in survival, cancer by cancer, that are meant to encourage researchers to look for more substantive improvements in the trials we run—so-called meaningful benefits.

Interestingly, the way expert oncologists use the phrase *meaningful benefit* in the biomedical literature falls short of this. My colleagues and I compared the benefits oncologists said were clinically meaningful in the academic literature against the ASCO and ESMO thresholds. We found that when academic oncologists called a PFS benefit meaningful, it met ASCO and ESMO thresholds 68% of the time. When they called an OS benefit meaningful, it met the threshold just 43% and 29% of the time, respectively.[17] Perhaps what is going on here is that some authors of biomedical studies seize upon any opportunity to hype drugs with limited benefits.

Who Should Design and Conduct Trials?

Ideally, the entire agenda for drug discovery trials would be set by nonconflicted parties. In the current system, a drug company decides what trial to conduct and presents the FDA with a report detailing the trial results. I think a better system would be using a nonconflicted group of academic experts to design and conduct randomized trials. Instead of a drug company coming to the FDA with a report of its own findings, the company should come with the drug in a bottle or bag, the preclinical data, and the amount of money it would otherwise spend on the phase 3 trial. Then the FDA, or a similar governmental body, would design and conduct the randomized trial.

In 2012, Adam Cifu, John Ioannidis, and I wrote the following in the *Journal of the American Medical Association:*

> Large trials of new innovations should be designed and conducted by investigators without conflicts of interest, under the auspices of non-conflicted scientific bodies. Instead of designing, controlling, and conducting the trials, manufacturers may offer the respective budget to a centralized public pool of funding, keeping the trial design and conduct independent. Asking corporate sponsors to conduct pivotal trials on their own products is like asking a painter to judge his or her own painting so as to receive an award. If a manufacturer can be allowed to manipulate the system to create a blockbuster product from an ineffective drug, the temptation is hard to resist.[18]

The need for a clinical trial agenda and drug approval agenda set by nonconflicted experts is greater than ever before.[19]

Can You Perform Randomized Controlled Trials of Rare Diseases?

The final topic we must discuss is how to handle a persistent objection to the importance of randomized trials in cancer medicine: can we conduct randomized trials for rare tumors with very low annual incidence?[20] At some point, there are not enough patients with a rare disease to study in a randomized trial, right?

First, as we discussed, one can be creative and use randomized trials to test strategies. For instance, if you want to pair patients with drugs in a truly individualized way, you can test the strategy of personalized oncology versus treating patients as you always had been (chapter 8). For now, though, let's put this aside and discuss another question. If we did want to generate data for a single rare tumor type, can it be done with a randomized trial?

It is worth noting that the FDA defines a rare or orphan disease as one that affects fewer than 200,000 people in the United States. That itself is fairly liberal, and many cancer types fall under this definition. Nevertheless, there are rare conditions, affecting fewer than 200,000 people, and then there are ultrarare conditions that may affect just hundreds of patients.

What's the rarest cancer for which we have randomized trials? If you want to appreciate the feasibility of randomization, it is useful to see exactly which rare cancers have had randomized trials done on them. To my knowledge, the rarest is adrenocortical cancer. The FIRM-ACT trial randomized over 300 patients to two different chemotherapy regimens. This tumor appears only in around one person per million,[21] where only 200 to 500 patients are diagnosed each year in the United States.[22] It is worth noting that the FIRM-ACT trial happened because researchers across the globe were willing to collaborate.

But how much rarer can a condition be before randomization becomes impossible? I concede that if a tumor is diagnosed in just a dozen patients globally per year, then a randomized trial becomes hard to imagine. Yet, we don't know the lower bound of randomization because randomization requires cooperation among academic doctors, which is difficult. One reason why doctors don't want to cooperate for a single randomized trial is that only one person can be the first listed author. Instead, if each pursued his or her own uncontrolled study, each can be first author on a paper. The phrase "publish or perish" still holds strong in the medical research field. FIRM-ACT is the rarest tumor for which we have randomization in 2018. One in a million is quite rare. Perhaps, with better networks and better collaboration, we can someday get down to one in 10 million. I don't know, but we should not be fatalists.

The last piece of data on randomization in rare cancers comes from the FDA itself. In 2012, the FDA reviewed its experience with rare cancers and drug approval. It noted that some cancers occur at rates of 6/100,000, others at 5/100,000, others at 4/100,000—you get the idea—down to 1/100,000. Keep in mind, a cancer that occurs in 1/100,000 is six times rarer than one that occurs in 6/100,000. Yet, the authors found that the percentage of trials that were randomized were 33% in the less than 6/100,000 group and 30% in the less than 1/100,000 group.[23] In other words, despite these cancers being six times rarer, randomization occurred at roughly the same rate as in less rare conditions. The fact that there was no detectable relationship between randomization and how rare a cancer was suggests that randomization, at least at these levels of rare, is feasible and can happen if researchers work together.

Conclusion

The current system has oversized incentives to get a single p-value of less than 0.05, and we have reached a point where it may even be profitable for drug companies to run trials on completely inert drugs. The likelihood that some will be positive by chance alone and the financial reward from this success could justify their entire portfolio. Of course, I don't think this is what is truly happening, but this incentive may explain why so many trials are conducted for drugs that are simply not promising, why the sample size of trials is growing steadily, and why approved drugs often have marginal benefits.

In an ideal world, active drugs will be pursued in randomized trials for regulatory approval. The trials would first be conducted in severe disease states and powered for meaningful overall survival benefits. These trials will be completed fast, because the event rate is unfortunately high in the severe disease state. It won't take long for a lifesaving drug to demonstrate efficacy (or effectiveness)* when patients are

---

* Efficacy is proof a therapy works under some ideal circumstances. Effectiveness is proof it works among patients in the real world.

dealing with terminal cancer. At the same time, if a drug does not help, the lack of benefit will be demonstrated early, not after society and patients have spent billions of dollars.

Next, drugs should be advanced to earlier disease states in trials that test them against giving the same drug in later disease states. Only such a trial asks the key question: is routine upfront use beneficial? Some may say that these trials will take too long, but they would only take a long time if moving the drug up does not greatly improve outcomes. If the drug is vital for patients, it will advance quickly. Trials should be designed by nonconflicted groups, who can be thoughtful about the comparator, doses, dose reduction, and population studied. Moreover, the moment the trial is halted by the monitoring committee because it demonstrated efficacy, the drug can be approved, as the trial was designed by regulators and will not then require their review. This may even speed approval.

Finally, this paradigm of drug development should be the rule and not the exception. Although I am sympathetic to the use of surrogates where there are truly no options, and although I concede that for some ultrarare conditions, this model will not fit, those are truly exceptional cases. Currently, the exceptions have become the rule, and oncology drug development is a mess. It is time to start mopping it up.

FOURTEEN

What Can Three Federal Agencies Do Tomorrow?

Good judgment is the result of experience and experience the result of bad judgment.
Mark Twain

MANY OF the issues raised in this book seem as if they are intractable or require political maneuvering to solve. It turns out that some of the challenges are difficult, requiring creative, perhaps even legislative, solutions, but it would be incorrect to believe there is nothing short of this we can do. In this chapter, I wish to outline specific things that three federal agencies can do tomorrow. Those agencies are the Food and Drug Administration (FDA), the Centers for Medicaid and Medicare Services (CMS), and the National Institutes of Health (NIH). All three have options at their disposal that could be immediately implemented, and improve the situation. And, there are additional fixes that can work over the longer term.

Things the FDA Can Do Tomorrow

The FDA is understandably defensive on the topic of "Could you be doing a better job?" In 2017, it tweeted the following from its professional account (fig. 14.1).[1] In the tweet,* the FDA says it does not set the standard of care, it doesn't set prices, and it cannot demand com-

---

* Now, you may be wondering, "Why are you citing Twitter and not a peer reviewed document?" For future readers, 2018 was a year in which the news cycle would often consist solely of covering one person's tweets. So, get off my case, and tell it to CNN.

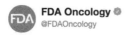

FDA Oncology ✔
@FDAOncology

Misconceptions about FDA: 1. We don't set standards of care. 2. We don't have anything to do w drug pricing. 3. We don't have comparative efficacy standard. Drugs don't have to be better than avail therapy- Pazdur #SABCS17

6:56 AM - 6 Dec 2017

34 Retweets **44** Likes

💬 2   🔁 34   ♡ 44   ✉

Figure 14.1. Tweet by @FDAOncology listing "misconceptions about the FDA"

parative trials. There is some truth in each of these statements, but at the same time it is half wrong. There are many actions the FDA has within its existing authority to make a positive impact on each of these fronts. Let's discuss the truth and then the fiction.

The FDA is charged with ensuring that the drugs that come to the market are safe and effective. It doesn't decide how medicine is practiced, and it is not the final arbiter of how drugs are used. Many drugs are used off-label, and some of that off-label use is good and necessary, while some is concerning and unsupported. The FDA doesn't tell doctors exactly when and how to give medications and in whom surgery or other unregulated procedures should be performed. This is the job of professional norms and guidelines.

Moreover, the FDA cannot force manufacturers to do head-to-head trials of contemporary drugs that work for similar indications or uses. This is called a *comparative effectiveness* authority, and the simple fact is that the US Congress, perpetually under heavy lobbying from the pharmaceutical industry, has never given the FDA that authority.

Finally, the FDA is right, it does not set drug prices, nor can it use price as a consideration in its decision making. It does not control how companies price medications. Thus, each of these three statements is technically correct, but in all three cases there are things the FDA can do that would (1) better inform the practice of medicine, (2) encourage trials that test novel drugs against the best existing therapies, and (3) lower prices. Let's start with trials comparing novel drugs to alternatives.

Ensuring Fair Comparisons without a Comparative Effectiveness Statute

While it is undeniable that the FDA does not set standard of care and cannot mandate comparative trials, it does have one power. It can halt trials that are blatantly and clearly unethical. It can't make you test your new cancer drug against another new cancer drug, but it can require you to test it against an accepted standard of care. It can strongly discourage companies from going abroad to a part of the world that is resource starved, where people may truly have no options, and test their fancy new drug against a placebo (chapter 12).

In 2018, in the *Lancet Oncology,* Derrick Tao and I gave four examples of clinical trials that led to FDA approval that used control arms inferior to the prevailing standards of care in the United States at the time of the study.[2] In all four cases, the FDA had the authority to demand a control arm in line with US standards. Let me summarize two of the cases here.

First, consider ibrutinib. On March 4, 2016, the FDA gave ibrutinib an expansive approval. Previously, the drug could only be used for people with chronic lymphocytic leukemia (CLL) as a second-line drug or if a patient had a specific mutation (17p loss).* The FDA allowed the company to broaden its indication to CLL, in general, including as initial therapy. This approval resulted in a substantial increase in market share, and the FDA granted it on the basis of a single randomized controlled trial called RESONATE-2.[3,4]

RESONATE-2 randomized 269 patients to either chlorambucil, an

---

* 17p is a genetic event that, in this case, identifies a group of patients with more aggressive cancer.

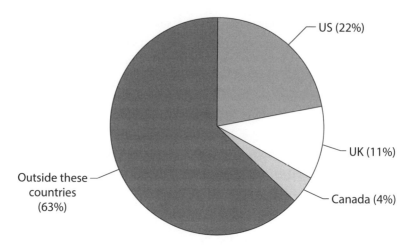

US (22%)

UK (11%)

Canada (4%)

Outside these
countries
(63%)

Figure 14.2. Locations of patients participating in the RESONATE-2 trial

old, cheap drug, or ibrutinib, the new, costly drug. Ibrutinib improved progression-free and overall survival, so the FDA approval of this drug seemed a natural extension of the findings. What's the problem then?

There are two problems with this. First, the trial was extensively conducted outside of the United States. Only 37% of patients came from the United States, United Kingdom, or Canada and just 22% from the United States (fig. 14.2). This matters because the standard of care after progression in many of these nations is dissimilar to that of the United States. For instance, one drug that was already available at progression in the United States, but essentially unavailable in many of these countries, was ibrutinib. Thus, we do not know if up-front ibrutinib improves survival over ibrutinib on the back end, which would be the relevant question for US citizens (see crossover in chapter 9).

The second problem is the control arm. Prior to this study, chlorambucil was rarely used in the United States, as it had already been beaten by several other drugs. In a devastating *New England Journal of Medicine* letter, Sharman and colleagues note, "Chlorambucil has served as a comparator in trials of bendamustine, alemtuzumab, ofatumumab, and obinutuzumab, and longer durations of progression-free survival have been reported with each agent." In other words, prior to this study, we already knew chlorambucil was inferior to alternatives.[5] The next point was even more damning. Sharman and colleagues studied their own United States–based CLL registry and found that only 4.5% of patients in the United States actually receive chlorambucil. Their conclusion: "Because of the superiority of alternative first-line regimens and the infrequent use of chlorambucil monotherapy, we do not think that chlorambucil monotherapy should serve as a comparator regimen in future studies of CLL."[5]

Chlorambucil should not have been used as the comparator for this registration study. It was seldom used in the United States and had been beaten by alternatives. Ibrutinib should have had to prove superiority to the therapies doctors were practically using, that is, the prevailing standard of care. By allowing the company to use chlorambucil, the FDA provided tacit support for an inferior control arm. Although the FDA lacks comparative effectiveness power, it does have the power to say, "Look, you can't go to countries that have standard of care inferior to the United States, test your drug against a straw man comparator, and then seek US approval claiming a survival advantage." The FDA could do this tomorrow but chooses not to.

Another example of a poor trial design that should have been rejected by the FDA is the trial for nivolumab. On December 22, 2014, the FDA approved nivolumab for metastatic melanoma. The approval was accelerated, although nivolumab had shown survival benefit over the control arm, dacarbazine, in a phase 3 randomized trial. What gives? If you have an OS benefit in a randomized trial, why would approval be accelerated and not regular?

First, a bit of background. Between 2006 and 2008, over 500 patients were randomized to dacarbazine, which was widely used in melanoma, plus placebo or dacarbazine plus ipilimumab, a new immunotherapy drug. In 2011, the trial was reported in the *NEJM,* showing a survival advantage with the combination of ipilimumab plus dacarbazine in patients with untreated metastatic melanoma. Then, two years later, nivolumab was tested against dacarbazine in over 500 patients in a trial that enrolled in Europe, Israel, Australia, Canada, and South America but not the United States. Why not the United States? Probably because no one would be willing to give a patient dacarbazine. The nivolumab versus dacarbazine trial was reported in the *NEJM* in November 2014.[6]

Let me summarize what happened here: years after we knew there was a better alternative to dacarbazine in metastatic melanoma, a trial was run testing a new drug against dacarbazine, and those results were used to seek approval in the United States, when not a single patient in that trial came from the United States.

Then, on December 22, 2014, the FDA gave approval for nivolumab using data from this randomized trial, but only the nivolumab arm. It gave the approval based on a "single-arm, non-comparative, planned interim analysis of the first 120 patients who received OPDIVO [nivolumab] in Trial 1 and in whom the minimum duration of follow up was 6 months" (page 14).[7] In other words, the FDA took a randomized trial, threw out the randomized part, and gave the approval—an accelerated approval—based on response rate. Reading between the lines, I wonder if the FDA was frustrated by this poor trial, but still was unwilling to lay down the law, and found a way to facilitate approval. Think back to chapter 6: if you knew there was a one in three or one in two chance you would someday be on the other side of the table, would you play hard ball?

Yet, instead of bending over backward to grant approval, the FDA could have, and should have, told the company that if you want regulatory approval in the United States, you have to do a randomized trial of nivolumab in the United States and test it against drugs that people are currently using in the United States. You cannot go abroad and conduct a trial testing nivolumab against an antiquated and defeated comparator. You might ask (but I hope you wouldn't, after reading the previous 13 chapters of this book): why not have the company conduct a single-arm, uncontrolled trial? I would argue that it would be insufficient in front-line melanoma, when current care was already guided by phase 3 data.

During the publication of this book, Talal Hilal, Mohamad Sonbol, and I decided to study this formally. We examined all FDA drug approvals between January 2013 and July 2018. We found that among 95 randomized studies leading to drug approval, 16 (17%) used a substandard control arm.[8] The concern raised here is part of a systematic problem.

The overall lesson is, while the FDA does not have comparative effectiveness authority, it does have the authority to halt unethical trials. A trial that tests a drug against a therapy already known to be inferior to alternatives is unethical. It is a straw man comparison. These tend to happen in poorer parts of the world, as we have seen in chapter 12. The FDA needs to stand up and say, "We will not accept these studies." Do that once and watch the industry retool its entire thinking.

Ensuring Appropriate Post-Protocol Therapy

In chapter 9, I discussed the important issue of crossover. You don't want it in trials assessing the fundamental efficacy of a novel drug, but it is a must in trials that seek to advance a drug that is already used in a later line of therapy.

As you can imagine, companies have lots of reasons to want to move a drug forward to the initial treatment of a condition—in many cases, they may have billions of reasons. The market share in the front-line, newly diagnosed or untreated cancer populations is generally much larger than the relapsed, refractory setting, both because more people face the former than the latter situation and because they take the drugs for longer periods of time. Yet, the key question in this situation is whether up-front use of the drug is superior to using the drug in a later line of therapy.

As I described in chapter 13, proper cancer drug development should show that drugs work (on patient-centered endpoints) in the last line and then gradually attempt to advance those drugs forward. To do this fairly, researchers must ensure that patients in the control arm receive the same drug upon progression. In other words, these trials should have crossover for the simple reason that using the drug upon progression reflects US standard of care.

One way companies appear to circumvent this policy is to conduct their trials in nations that do not have that drug available at all. Now, before I give you examples, let me make one thing clear. This type of bias—unfair post-protocol therapy—will not impact the first progression or PFS (that is, before patients would receive these drugs), but it will affect the second progression, third progression, and overall survival. As I argued in chapter 10, when you move drugs earlier in therapy, you have to improve overall survival.

Consider the case of bortezomib in mantle cell lymphoma. In 2014, the FDA approved bortezomib, a new and costly drug, for the up-front treatment of mantle cell lymphoma. Bortezomib was approved in a combo called VR-CAP[9] (the "V" is for bortezomib, or Velcade). VR-CAP beat R-CHOP (rituximab plus CHOP; chapter 9) in a global trial based on a superior PFS and overall survival.[10] What's the problem?

The problem is that bortezomib was already approved by the FDA as a salvage treatment for mantle cell lymphoma in the United States for relapsed patients. In this fashion, bortezomib was widely used in the United States, but because of price, was not available throughout much of the world. So the critical question in 2014—the question that the FDA should have compelled the manufacturer to answer—was not whether VR-CAP is better than R-CHOP. It was: is VR-CAP better than R-CHOP, when patients who progress on R-CHOP have access to bortezomib?

Yet, in the VR-CAP trial, patients were recruited from 128 centers across 28 countries on four continents. Only 7% of patients got bortezomib as a subsequent therapy[11] after receiving and progressing on R-CHOP. VR-CAP may have a better PFS than R-CHOP, but would it have improved OS if patients getting R-CHOP were allowed to get bortezomib later? Unless the control arm gets the same standard of care postprogression as in the United States, we cannot know this for sure. Here, too, the FDA can raise regulatory standards. The FDA can refuse to approve drugs conducted in settings globally where post-protocol care is beneath US standard. It can simply say, "If you are seeking US approval, you need to use US standard of care post-protocol." It might even add a pro tip: you could conduct your trial in the USA to make that easy.

I am just going to give one more example here, although I could go on and on. This is one where I suspect that the drug does have benefit, but as tested, it has a poor value—in other words, a high dollar-per-life-year added. Had it been tested correctly, it would be even higher.

Do you remember back in chapter 1 when I said pertuzumab, an anti-HER2 drug, in breast cancer costs $473,000 to add a single life-year? That was based on a cost-effectiveness paper,[12] which assumed the drug added 15.7 months of median survival. That was a fair assumption because it was exactly what was seen in the CLEOPATRA trial,[13] which randomized patients receiving trastuzumab and a taxane with either placebo or pertuzumab. However, a key limitation to this trial was what happened after patients progressed. Only 68% of patients received trastuzumab (or other HER2-directed therapy) after progression. That percentage is simply not what would happen if this trial were solely conducted in the United States. In the United States, 100% (or nearly that) would have received HER2-directed drugs.

In the United States, we have three HER2-directed treatment options upon progression: more trastuzumab, T-DM1, or lapatinib, with several trials supporting each of them and some showing survival benefit. In other words, how much of the 15-month benefit is due to pertuzumab and how much is due to the control arm doing worse because the patients did not receive US standard of care?* Had the trial been conducted with US standards, I suspect (but cannot prove) the benefit would be slightly smaller, and the cost-effectiveness slightly poorer, though I still think the drug would have succeeded.

Slowing Duplicative Drugs

The FDA does not have comparative effectiveness authority, but it is also under no obligation to repeatedly approve similar drugs in the exact same indication based on uncontrolled data. Here, too, it can say no.

Consider bladder cancer. For the treatment of bladder cancer that has progressed after initial therapy, we have five approved options (as

---

* Poor post protocol therapy here is not crossover to the investigational agent, but nevertheless will disproportionately affect the control arm because more patients come off study and require further treatment. I am putting this as a footnote because it is a complicated point that it is not important for all to understand.

of June 2017) that inhibit PD1 or PDL1, a key immunology check-point. Those drugs are: atezolizumab (approved May 18, 2016, based on a single-arm trial); nivolumab (approved February 2, 2017, based on a single-arm trial); durvalumab (approved May 1, 2017, based on a single-arm trial); avelumab (approved May 9, 2017, based on single-arm trial data); and pembrolizumab (approved May 18, 2017, based on randomized data that showed that it led to better survival than chemotherapy).

What is going on? Of course, most of us would agree that we don't need five next-in-class drugs for the same purpose unless the cost is lower. Spoiler alert: it isn't. The FDA says that it has no comparative effectiveness power so it cannot force these manufacturers to compare their drugs. Yet, the FDA could decide that only one PD1 drug can gain accelerated approval based on response rate here. Unless you present a drug with a dramatically better response rate, you must now come to the table with randomized data showing a survival benefit. The unmet need that existed—and we can debate whether it existed*—is now closed. Feel free to approve atezolizumab based on uncontrolled data, but nivolumab, durvalumab, and avelumab no longer fill an unmet need and can be declined. Pembrolizumab, of course, has randomized data on overall survival and can secure a regular approval.

Patients Who Look Like Americans

As I have discussed, the age of patients in FDA trials is far below the average age of cancer patients in the United States. In other ways, patients on trials are healthier and have fewer medical problems than the average cancer patient. As just one example, in chapter 1 I discussed how few Kaiser Permanente patients were eligible for contemporary trials.

---

* You may find it blasphemous that I ask whether the unmet need existed, since chemotherapy in second-line bladder cancer is not terrific. A few thoughts: first, the trials in this setting did not compare immunotherapy to pemetrexed and nab-paclitaxel, which had the strongest single-arm data; and second, the response rate of immunotherapy is around 5%–10% better than chemotherapy. Given the side effect profile, I am willing to concede that immunotherapy is better, but not much better.

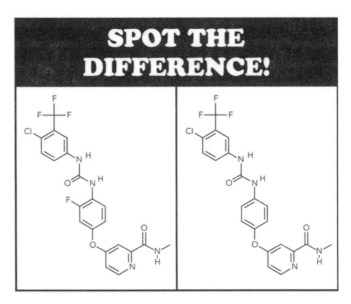

Figure 14.3. Me-too drugs. Comparing sorafenib with regorafenib. Can you see the subtle difference? Used with permission by *Nature Reviews Clinical Oncology.*

We must remember that the FDA exists to regulate the US drug and device industry for its citizens, not the idealized patients. The FDA can and should deny approval for drugs that are tested in patients who look nothing like average patients. It will only take a few whacks of the ruler before we would rapidly see a change in clinical trials moving toward enrolling representative Americans.

I would start with regorafenib.[14] Regorafenib is a next-in-class, or a me-too, drug that bears a close resemblance, chemically, to sorafenib. In fact, the resemblance is striking (fig. 14.3). Sorafenib gained FDA approval for hepatocellular carcinoma based on a trial in 2007 called SHARP. I discussed sorafenib in chapter 1. There, I made the point that the real-world data for this drug was sobering. Although the drug appeared to add about three months of survival in the pivotal trial (from 8 to 11 months), in the real world, it doesn't seem to add any time (in a propensity score–matched analysis), and patients treated with the drug in the real world did worse than patients who received supportive care in the clinical trial.

A few years later, regorafenib was shown in trials to be better than supportive care for patients who progressed on sorafenib. The trial had bizarre inclusion criteria: patients "must have tolerated sorafenib (≥400 mg daily for at least 20 of the 28 days before discontinuation) and received their last sorafenib dose within 10 weeks of randomization. They were required to have Child-Pugh A liver function. Patients were excluded if they . . . Discontinued [because of] sorafenib . . . toxicity."[15]

Where do I begin? The regorafenib trial led to FDA approval, but it was far worse than the usual unrepresentative trial because the usual unrepresentative trial merely includes younger patients with fewer comorbidities than the average American. This trial does more. First, you had to have taken sorafenib to be eligible to receive the trial drug. This itself removes the sick patients.

Second, you had to have tolerated sorafenib, which is hard to do for 20 out of 28 days. This removes more sick patients. You had to have excellent liver function. You could not have stopped the prior therapy for toxicity. In the supplement, the authors add that you have to have a life expectancy of at least three months! All removing more and more patients.

Data suggest that only 27% of Americans with metastatic liver cancer actually get sorafenib.[16] Data from a Taiwanese registry show[17] that, at most, 30% of patients might be considered for another therapy after sorafenib. This means that, at best, regorafenib will benefit 8% of liver cancer patients. However, the true percentage is likely even lower, given the severe restrictions on who could enter the trial.

If you work at the FDA, you have to lay down the law. If trial participants don't look like the average person in the United States, then restrict the approval to the patient qualities (age, cancer stage, and so on) studied. Restrict the approval to the inclusion criteria of the study, or flatly deny the approval. If the FDA does it once or twice, the entire industry will retool. Instead, the approval for regorafenib makes no mention of needing to progress on sorafenib while taking it diligently and remaining free of notable side effects, all while remaining fit.

Surrogate Endpoints

I discussed this extensively in chapters 2 and 3, but the FDA could actually enforce statutory language around the use of surrogate endpoints. Regular approval should be reserved for surrogates only if they are validated in trial-level analyses. Accelerated approval should be granted only in situations where there is truly an unmet need, that is, cancers that are dire, rare, and with truly no treatment options. Postmarketing efficacy requirements showing survival benefit must be the norm in these cases.

One of the persistent arguments the FDA makes for why it is heavily reliant on surrogates is that the response rate of drugs is often so high that equipoise is lost—meaning that no reasonable oncologist or patient would be randomized to a placebo. The response rate is so high, the drug must work, the logic goes. Yet, as we saw in chapter 11 with Iodine 131-tositumumab, a drug can have a high response rate but still fail to improve outcomes. But more to the point, the FDA is approving drugs based on response rates that are generally modest. Led by Emerson Chen, we found that the median response rate among drugs that are approved based on response rate is 41%, and the median complete response rate is 6%.[18] Contrast that with drugs that are truly transformative. Remember in chapter 1, imatinib had nearly a 100% complete response rate in its phase 1 trial. Most drugs approved based on response are no imatinib.

Finally, all accelerated approvals should have to show they improve survival or quality of life after these drugs come to the market. As we saw in chapter 3, the FDA has a poor track record with enforcing these commitments. The FDA should set time limits (for example, five years) and enforce them strictly, revoking the approval of companies that fail to deliver. Finally, the FDA cannot use the same surrogate to convert accelerated approvals to regular approvals. This may sound obvious, but it is an actual problem. Researchers from Harvard found that 37% of the time the FDA converts accelerated approvals to regular approvals based on trials that measure the same surrogate endpoint, and not survival or quality of life.[19] Needless to say, this defies common sense. If the surrogate was only "reasonably likely to predict" at the outset, measuring it a second time does not provide assurance that the drug actually helps people with cancer live longer or better lives.

Minimum Benefit

The final solution that the FDA could implement tomorrow was proposed by Justin Bekelman and Steven Joffe of the University of Pennsylvania. These authors note that the FDA already has the regulatory authority to define the size of benefit that warrants approval. This could easily be strengthened into setting clinically meaningful benefits.[20] For instance, 10-day survival gain for pancreatic cancer is likely too small to truly matter to patients. Setting realistic, modest minimum benefits would encourage the industry to pursue more innovative drugs. It may even reduce the sample size and cost of clinical trials. Already both the American Society of Clinical Oncology and the European Society of Medical Oncology have proposed guidelines, tumor by tumor, for what constitutes meaningful benefit. This proposal could be implemented immediately.

Legislative Solutions

The above solutions are course corrections that I think the FDA could take in the absence of legislative changes, but true solutions might require Congress to pass a bill to reform the FDA.

Based on the themes I have explored, the low-hanging fruit is to grant the FDA formal comparative effectiveness authority. This would permit the agency to demand that drugs in the pipeline are tested against one another. But, if you are going to fix the situation legislatively, you can think big. A fundamental solution here is: move the design and conduct of clinical trials from companies to an impartial agency (as discussed in chapter 13). It doesn't have to be the FDA, but it should be a federally funded agency that utilizes nonconflicted consultants (for example, patients, doctors, methodologists without industry ties) as voting members. Conflicted experts could provide verbal input but have no voting power. This nonconflicted group would be charged with the design, conduct, and reporting of trials for drug approval. In the current system, we allow the pharma company to design and conduct a study, which is often low quality, and then presents the FDA with the study report, along with a several-million-dollar drug application fee. Instead, why not have the company submit its compound, preclinical data, early phase data, and a sum of money to cover the trial?

There are many advantages to this proposal. First, the group designing the trial would have already vetted and validated it, so if the trial generates a positive result, approval can happen immediately. This would have the benefit of drugs coming to market faster—300 days faster than the current system.[21] In other words, we won't need the FDA to review the trial design on the back end; it will have consented to the trial design on the front end.

Second, nonconflicted experts can decide how and against what to test the drug product. In the case of bladder cancer, this would ensure that when five PD1/PDL1 drugs are coming to market with early phase data, they are tested against each other, and perhaps we could actually learn, sometime this century, which is best.

Third, trials can be powered to detect clinically meaningful benefits. These won't be trials looking for survival benefits measured in days. These trials would be looking for substantive benefits for patients. At a minimum, guidance from American and European professional societies can be used.

Fourth, the choice of patients, control/comparison arm, dose, and post-protocol therapy will all be designed to reflect the US patient population. Unlike the sponsor, the nonconflicted expert body will be tasked with optimizing trials for the US population.

Fifth, the sponsor need not be excluded and can participate as a nonvoting member of the discussion. Both the industry and conflicted experts may lend their voices, but the final vote should be made by only those without conflict. Moreover, testimony can be sought from prominent academic groups who think deeply about trial methodology. Elsewhere in this book (chapter 7), I have suggested more experts become nonconflicted. The way to make this happen is to continue to insert disincentives to becoming conflicted, as this would be. Ultimately, experts in methods and clinical trials should be the final arbiters of which trials are worth pursuing.*

Some may be concerned that the FDA will drag its heels and not run trials quickly. Nevertheless, the FDA has proved it can meet strict deadlines in getting drugs approved. There is no reason to doubt, with sufficient resources, it can meet trial deadlines as well.

Of course, my proposal would not stop other parties from running trials. The best policy solutions gently redirect the system. Cooperative groups and federally funded research can continue to test drugs and devices, as they do now.

What Can the CMS Do?

Before I tell you what the Centers for Medicare and Medicaid Services (CMS) should do, let's take a moment to review how bad the current state of affairs has become. Through a quirk of legislation, the CMS cannot negotiate price. It must pay for every FDA-approved therapy. Finally, it must also pay for any medication recommended for off-label use by one of several expert guideline bodies or compendia, including that of the NCCN (discussed in chapter 6).

Your first question might be why? Why would the CMS pay for a drug recommended off-label at all? Let me start by saying that originally this made some sense. In the late 1980s and early 1990s, the majority of cancer drugs were cytotoxic and relatively cheap. In many cases, patents had expired and these drugs were generic. Doctors used these drugs in a variety of cancers, but the drug did not always have FDA approval. Nevertheless, sometimes there were strong data. Since these drugs were old and cheap, there was little incentive for any company to seek a formal FDA approval, as such, much of the use was

---

* For more discussion of this topic, read this: http://www.bmj.com/content/345/bmj .e7031.

off-label, and the guidelines provided some record of what was reasonable or not. Fast-forward 25 years, and the situation was different. Most new anticancer drugs cost in excess of $100,000 per year. These drugs are often branded (on patent), and the manufacturers have tremendous incentive and ability to seek subsequent FDA approvals. Thus, a system designed at a time when drugs were cheap is being applied at a time where drugs cost a fortune—and that may no longer make sense.

In 2017, my colleagues and I studied the NCCN recommendations broadly. We wanted to know: How often does the NCCN recommend FDA approved therapies, and how often does it go beyond the FDA approvals? When it extrapolates beyond the FDA, what sort of evidence does it provide?[22]

We looked at 47 drugs that had been granted 69 FDA approvals. All 69 approvals were included in the NCCN guidelines. So far, so good. But what surprised us was that another 44 additional uses or extrapolations were provided by the NCCN. In other words, 39% of NCCN recommendations are extrapolations or went beyond the FDA approvals.

Next, we asked ourselves what was the level of data provided. The most common source of data was . . . "no data provided," which accounted for 36% of recommendations, and only 16% were based on randomized controlled trials. In short, the NCCN often expanded recommendations beyond what was approved by the FDA based on low levels of data. This might be fine were it not for the fact that the authors of this guideline are heavily conflicted (see chapter 6), and the report mandates that the CMS pay for these drugs. The CMS is essentially being compelled to pay for drugs with little to no cited data.

The solution here is simple. The CMS should replace the NCCN with its own compendia. It can solicit input from nonconflicted oncologists and develop its own guidelines. It should not be compelled to pay for drugs recommended based on little data by a group of oncologists who are on the pharmaceutical payroll.

With a reformed FDA, the job of the CMS will be easier. If the drugs that come to market offer better benefits on average, the CMS will be more comfortable paying. The CMS should be given the authority to use cost-effectiveness to pursue a fair price and to negotiate freely. It must be given the right to say no. If the design and conduct of cancer trials moves to nonconflicted groups, the need to say no would likely happen less and less, as the drugs that do make it to the market will offer meaningful benefits.

What Can the NIH Do?

Although I stated at the outset that this is not a cancer biology book, overcoming the biology of cancer is the key to developing effective therapies. While successful science is hard to predict, and insights often occur through serendipitous and unexpected routes,[23] there are some policy initiatives we could implement that may help scientific progress against cancer. Here I will outline three ideas: consistent, growing science funding, testing grant funding, and implementing a nonconflicted clinical trials portfolio.

The amount of money used to fund cancer biology research is a tiny fraction of the economic and human cost of the disease. Although the US National Cancer Institute receives an annual budget of $5 billion, this is likely not enough spending on cancer biology research for the simple reason that the economic toll of cancer and the amount we spend on cancer care is two orders of magnitude larger. I would propose steady, incremental growth in cancer research funding. Growth must be ensured over time, through different government cycles or changing political priorities. Some portion of the budget should go toward "blue sky" science, or science performed solely with the goal of better understanding how the world works. The current environment is punishing for cancer biology researchers. The median age of receiving R01 funding, a career milestone, is creeping upward now nearing 50 years of age (45 for one's first R01).[24] Opportunities for careers in science research at universities are so few in comparison to the number of PhD graduates that some have called the system a "Ponzi scheme."[25] For this reason, a large, sustained increase in funding could draw more and younger scientists into studying cancer.

For the portion of science that is not blue sky but rather goal-directed or translational, the way we give out grant funding is suboptimal. Grants are not necessarily given to the authors of highly influential science,[26] and some data suggest that a handful of researchers who are extremely well funded are subject to diminishing returns.[27] In other words, a few scientists consume a large portion of grants and don't produce more as a result. The truth is that, as with any complex social and systemic challenge, no one knows the solution with certainty. Any proposal may have unintended and unanticipated effects. In situations like this the best path forward is the same as with unproven drugs or procedures—conduct randomized trials. John Ioannidis has proposed a number of alternatives to the current funding system, including performing a lottery, or funding more researchers by making grants smaller in size.[28] There is no need to speculate which of these might be best. We can actively experiment among alternative funding strategies and track outcomes, including measures of productivity and impact.

Finally, the third reform at the level of the NIH is to establish a nonconflicted trials agenda. This would go beyond the previously mentioned proposal at the FDA, and allocate substantial funding (for example, 2% to 5% of federal health care spending) on the establishment of such a program. These dollars can be used to test countless, clinically relevant questions that challenge doctors and patients daily. We spend approximately a trillion dollars on health care, and much of that spending is on interventions for which we truly do not know if patients benefit (for a full discussion of that topic read my prior coauthored book *Ending Medical Reversal*). A large, federally supported trials agenda would be able to address these questions, as well as issues of drug sequence or dosing that are simply forever unresolved in the current world. As with the other reforms, the budget for this agency should start low, but have slow, sustained, and consistent growth.

Conclusion

There are both short-term and long-term changes that can be made to the FDA, the CMS, and the NIH to encourage the pursuit, development, and marketing of transformational cancer drugs at more afford-able prices. I focused more of my attention on the FDA because I think it plays a more important role in this space. If cancer drug develop-ment was incentivized to pursue better agents, the decision to pay for these drugs would be easier. Ultimately, the argument that there is nothing we can do falls short. Existing regulatory language could em-power many solutions if we as a society were willing to pursue it.

FIFTEEN

What Can People with Cancer Do?

Give me six hours to chop down a tree and I will spend the first four sharpening the axe.

ABRAHAM LINCOLN

IN THE previous two chapters, I provided an outline of how drug development should proceed and made specific recommendations for what the FDA and CMS could do to ensure that cancer drug policy worked on behalf of people with cancer. Many of those suggestions were far reaching, and while some could be instituted tomorrow, the effects of most of them would materialize only on the order of years, as the entire system of drug development rearranges itself around them. In the meantime, what can cancer patients do to ensure that more of their care is in line with their goals and preferences? In this chapter, I will provide specific recommendations for patients who are referred to oncology.

The First Visit

People seeing an oncologist should have an understanding of their specific situation. Are you being referred for a suspicious blood test or mass? Is the diagnosis uncertain? Alternatively, has a cancer diagnosis been made? In your own mind, the reason why you are seeing the cancer specialist should be clear. If not, that's the first question you should ask.

If a cancer diagnosis has been made, there are some things you must learn on the first visit. What's the name of my condition? If I wanted to read about the topic, what should I look up (for example, disease, risk category, or stage)? Do I require treatment or is observation best? What additional studies are needed to decide upon treatment?

If treatment is advised, then you should understand whether the goal of that treatment is to cure the cancer or merely to slow its growth (palliative). It's important to be clear whether the goal of treatment is palliative or curative. If more information is needed to give the answer, then follow up later with your physician.

I would generally advise that the first visit with a cancer doctor is not the best time to discuss prognosis. It helps to have a relationship with the physician and trust him or her before broaching this subject. At the same time, prognosis is important, and when the topic does arise (usually on the second or third visit), I always recommend asking for ranges, rather than absolute numbers. Ranges convey what happens to most patients.

The Diagnosis

It's important to know how you were diagnosed with cancer. If it was a biopsy, obtain a copy of the report. Ask your doctor how sure he or she is in the diagnosis. How reliable are the pathologists? It is not always necessary, but also not unreasonable, to ask for the slides to be sent for a second review, particularly at a nearby academic medical hospital. If there is uncertainty, this is a must.

Scans

I would always advise patients to save a copy of their scan report and obtain a CD if possible. All information in the patient chart belongs to you. It is yours, and you might as well have a copy because someday it may come in handy. If you see a different physician, take these reports with you, but make sure you get them back before you leave.

Treatment

The most important time in the early visits is the discussion around treatment. A savvy patient can ask many questions to ensure the recommendation is in line with his or her preferences and goals. First, you should ask the tough question. What happens if I do nothing? Has anyone ever chosen that? Next, you need to clarify whether the goal of treatment is curative or palliative. Is it to get rid of the cancer forever or merely slow its growth? This is a fair time to ask about prognosis with or without treatment.

In my experience, patients immediately gravitate to the logistics of therapy—how often do I have to come in? This is an important question and must be addressed, but first try to understand the physician's reasoning about the choice of treatment. Ask what alternatives could be used. Why does the physician not favor those choices? If the physician is stuck—cannot name an alternative—ask what the treatment was in the years prior to the current regimen. Or ask what 100 different oncologists might say.

Why does the physician believe the proposed treatment is preferable? Can he or she explain it? Now is the time to utilize the skills from this book. Don't settle for mechanistic reasons. It isn't enough to get a lesson on cancer biology. One wants to know the data. What are the studies that support the logic of the proposed treatment? How and why is it superior to alternatives? What are the costs and toxicities?

Now is the time to talk about logistics. How often do I have to come in? Where do I go? How will I get my home medication? Can you provide me with a calendar of my visits? The list goes on and on, but you should be able to visualize what you need to do.

Second Opinions

Family, friends, and patients ask me when the right time is to get a second opinion, if at all. My answer is that it is never wrong to get a second opinion, but the best moments would be prior to starting the proposed treatment at diagnosis, and at the major treatment junctions, such as if the cancer progresses. It is important to press the doctor you see to go beyond answering the question: what should I do? Rather, a doctor should explain why he or she recommends one treatment versus an alternative. Of course, the most important thing about a doctor is finding someone you can trust.

On Therapy

While taking anticancer drugs, you should know how often and with what method the physician plans to assess your cancer. Will we use blood tests or CT scans? How often will we do them? If the plan involves repeat MRIs or PET CTs, it is always worth asking whether that particular intervention is necessary, or whether a plain ole CT might suffice.

Side Effects

It is important to report any side effects you may be having and ask what ways there might be to ameliorate them. It's easy to add more medications, but the same questions apply: Where is the evidence that shows they help? What are the alternatives? It's important to have a card listing all the medications you are taking and what the rationale is for each. Keep copies and keep it up to date.

Balancing Efficacy and Side Effects

If you are in the situation where the treatment you are receiving is palliative (not curative), then you should not forget that every day or month that you continue receiving the medication, you are making a calculation. Is the potential upside of this drug or therapy worth the downsides? There is no one-size-fits-all answer here, and you should be empowered to broach this question with your physician. Keep a log of your symptoms. Consider that just because you started a therapy does not obligate you to any duration of it. The choice is always yours, and you should be able to speak freely with your oncologist about your feelings.

Maintenance and Extending Therapy

In this book, I have argued that the bar for extending therapy ought to be improvements in overall survival. Yet, I respect that individuals may have a range of feelings on this topic. If your oncologist proposes putting you on maintenance therapy, ask to have more of a discussion about it. What can you read to better inform your choice?

Should I Participate in Clinical Trials?

Contrary to some in oncology, I cannot endorse every single trial out there. But, I can say that if you have the opportunity to participate in a randomized trial in cancer medicine run by a national cooperative group or other impartial body, you should seriously consider it. These are trials that answer pressing, practical questions in oncology and are being run precisely because we do not know the right answer. Lest you worry about the possibility of being assigned to an arm containing placebo, remember the old Thomas Chalmers quote, "One has only to review the graveyard of discarded therapies to discover how many patients might have benefited from being randomly assigned to a control group."

Don't Fall for Bioplausibility

It is worth restating this point: don't fall for bioplausibility; you need to hear data. If you ask your doctor, why are you giving me nivolumab? The wrong answer is because the drug unleashes the immune system. The right answer is because the drug was superior to the chemotherapy, the previously used treatment, in a randomized trial.

Don't Cling to Anecdotes

I hope that I have made the case that it is not useful to make sense of your situation from the most dramatic or unrepresentative anecdotes (see chapter 8). At the same time, I appreciate those who think the median does not capture everything you need to know. Instead, I advise you to ask doctors to give the 25th and 75th percentiles, or 20th and 80th, to provide a reasonable range of what you might expect. Again, not every patient will fall into such a range, but the majority of people will. And knowing this range allows you to hope for the best while preparing for the worst.

Alternative or Complementary Interventions

I am often asked whether or not I think an alternative or complementary therapy—such as CBD or mistletoe or curcumin or yoga or turmeric—will be helpful. The answer is usually that I have no knowledge of that intervention. My general approach is to say as long as a complementary therapy does not interfere with what we are doing, is not too expensive, and does not have serious downsides or contraindications, it is reasonable for people to do what they think is best.

Eating, Drinking, and Exercising

Patients often ask me what my advice is regarding eating, drinking, and exercising. Here, too, I strike a middle ground. I am not aware of any superfoods, magic teas, or rejuvenating exercises, but at the same time I don't favor any prohibitions. I think people should be free to do what they can tolerate and feels good. I encourage most patients to eat what they enjoy and to doubt that any severe restrictions (which seem more and more popular these days) are of substantial benefit. Many of the studies in this space are sadly as bad as the nuts study from chapter 9.

After Treatment

Whether your treatment is curative or palliative, there may come a moment when the doctor recommends halting therapy. In these cases, it is important to ask how we will monitor for recurrence of the cancer. Will we use scans or blood tests or a physical exam? What are the chances the cancer comes back? If recurrence is certain, what is the range of time people go before it returns?

For some cancers, the therapy was curative in intent. This means that at some point, a doctor will likely recommend no further scans and that the cancer is no more likely to return in you than someone who never had this cancer. In this situation, you should ask about the future and the long-term health risks from the treatment. Is there something you can do to mitigate that risk?

Talk to Family, Friends, and Loved Ones

My final piece of advice is that any diagnosis of cancer provides an opportunity to take stock of one's life. Who do you wish you spoke with more? Who do you want to visit? Spend time with people you love whether your cancer is life-threatening or not. In fact, it is something we should all do more often.

If your cancer is incurable, it's good to discuss your wishes around end-of-life care. It's important to appoint a power of attorney and medical decision maker. And, you should also communicate with those close to you who are not your decision maker, to avoid any confusion later.

End of Life

For too many patients, cancer, unfortunately, will result in their death. For patients receiving treatments that will not cure the disease, it's important to ask your doctor if a referral to a palliative care doctor may be appropriate. Palliative care doctors are experts who specialize in improving the symptoms for patients with chronic or terminal illnesses. They will likely help you clarify if the medications you are taking—and may have been taking for years—are still appropriate. Can you stop your statin medication, for instance?

Although I have championed better evidence throughout this book, I believe that much of end-of-life care can be based on common sense. Stopping a statin is one example that provides an interesting observation about our profession. The statin class of medication is one that lowers low-density lipoprotein and in many groups of patients, particularly those who have previously had a heart attack, these drugs can lower the rate of subsequent heart attacks or strokes. Of course, they are also used widely to improve cholesterol for patients who have not experienced problems, but with the hope the drug will reduce the risk of these events. People from both groups of patients may someday develop terminal cancer, and, largely through inertia, they remain on statin medications.

In 2015, a randomized trial was published that suggested it might be safe to stop statins in this group. The authors randomized 381 patients to either continue or discontinue their statin and had a primary endpoint of overall survival[1] at 60 days. Kaplan-Meier curves were largely superimposable. But, here's the problem. They ran this study as a noninferiority trial. And like many other NI trials (see chapter 11), they picked a large delta—a 5% absolute increase in death at 60 days. But because their sample size was small, and the fact that patients in this study lived longer than expected in both groups,* they found stopping statins was "not non-inferior." Although the authors spun their results to say that stopping statins was probably fine, some pedantic readers called them out on it.[2] Not non-inferior means you can't say for sure it is safe to stop, they counseled.

When I read this study, and the letter, I was shocked. What was going on? To my knowledge, no one had ever tested, nor proven, that statins improve outcomes for people with terminal cancer—which really is the only reason why you would take a medication: it provides a tangible benefit. Moreover, the majority of statin trials explicitly excluded patients with terminal cancer—thus the use of the statin medication group in these patients is absolutely unsupported. Moreover, it defies common sense that a patient should take a long-acting cardiovascular risk-modifying drug when faced with a lethal and terminal cancer. The only questions I was left with were: Did we need this study? Do we

---

* It is worth noting that a lower than expected event rate also reduces the power to conclude that non-inferiority is met.

really need non-inferiority trials to show that we can stop statin drugs in the terminally ill?

The mere fact that we conducted this study provides some clue that physicians have a hard time stopping therapy. If it is so difficult to persuade doctors to consider stopping statins, can you imagine how challenging it might be to suggest that perhaps we stop anticancer drugs? And yet, this is the situation many patients find themselves in. Sick and vulnerable and not sure when to focus on comfort. I think it is important to recognize that some in the medical profession and some oncologists might need a nudge from palliative doctors and patients when the time is right. Patients should feel comfortable having an open discussion with their doctor on this issue. It is never a wrong time to bring up the topic.

Lend Our Voice to the Public Debate

The final suggestion I have, and one thing all people can do, is lend their voice to the public debate. Every few years, Congress passes legislation regarding the FDA. Often, the newspaper headline sounds good. For instance, of course the FDA should approve drugs based on real-world data. What's the alternative? Unreal data? But a deeper understanding would lead you to know that real-world data are misused to mean nonrandomized data, and that would mean marked uncertainty about drugs that come to market. Similarly, a bill like "right to try" sounds good, because after all, who wants to stop someone from trying? But a deeper understanding would reveal that the bill bypasses the FDA's customary review for investigational drugs that have not yet proven their worth and may prey upon the hopes of desperate patients. Moreover, the bill does not address the real barriers to "trying," as the FDA grants 99% of requests currently, and companies are usually the ones denying requests.[3]

Conclusion

My advice is that you should engage in the political process. Understand health policy bills as deeply as possible, and use your voice to communicate your desires. Speak out for policies that lower drug prices. Ask for better standards of evidence. Don't be satisfied with billion-dollar drugs coming to the market based on surrogates and then not generating credible data for a decade or longer. One of the great threats to sound cancer policy is that a small and vocal minority can easily overrule a large and uninterested majority. In cancer medicine, because of the sums of money at stake and the intricacies of the issue, it is easy for the industry to advance its agenda, while citizens of this country may be uninterested, uninformed, and none-the-wiser. In fact, the deep prerequisite to all of the problems in this book is that our system has evolved to serve the interests of a few vocal groups who reap tremendous profits. It must be realigned to serve the interests of patients, the public, and society.

SIXTEEN

What Can Students, Residents, and Fellows Do?

The man who does not read books has no advantage over the man that cannot read them.

MARK TWAIN

I WANTED to end this book with an optimistic note, and there is nothing that gives me more optimism than the rising generation of students, residents, and fellows—a group that I collectively call "trainees." I consider trainees broadly. I hope to address anyone who aspires to be a hematologist oncologist, radiation oncologist, surgical oncologist, or a member of any other field of medicine with significant contact with cancer patients, including oncology pharmacists, social workers, and cancer counselors. Anyone who is on the path to be a health professional working largely with cancer patients can play an important role in the years to come. In this chapter, I give specific recommendations for what trainees can do.

Keeping Up with the Literature—By Yourself

Perhaps there was once a day when everything you needed to know for the job was learned in your training, and your career was merely the practice and refinement of that art. Unfortunately, that day is not 2020. In the modern cancer world, we are continually inundated with new information, some of which is indeed practice changing.

Keeping up with this information is no easy task, and in the course of a busy week, the temptation is to do so in the easiest way possible:

that is, glance at the free trade-publications mailed to you, attend local Continuing Medical Education (CME) activities, go to drug dinners when invited, and meet with drug company representatives who visit your office. I want to suggest that you don't do any of this.

Even if what you hear passively in these activities is factual, it may nevertheless be misleading because the curator of that information may be a for-profit entity that wants to direct your attention to its products. The passive way of keeping up with oncology will capture the most valuable thing in oncology education—your attention—and move it preferentially to topics that the speaker wants you to think about.

Instead, you should become the curator of the information you digest. Here is my proposal on how to do this. First, make a list of the key publications in your field. For me, it might be the *Journal of the American Medical Association (JAMA): Oncology* or the *Journal of Clinical Oncology (JCO)*. Find out when new articles are posted online. *JAMA: Oncology* generally arrives on Thursday, while the *JCO* comes in a continuous trickle. It pays to know when new articles come out because, in the hours and days afterward, a discussion will be taking place, one that you should take part in (more to come).

Next, every time new articles are released, go to the website and scan the titles. Look for topics and titles that interest you—that concern your practice. For ones that make your cut (for me maybe one in four), skim the abstract. Think back to chapter 9. Which articles are worth a deep dive? As a general rule, nonrandomized, small sample size, surrogate endpoint studies, are less enticing than randomized, prospective, multicenter trials measuring survival or quality of life. Don't set hard and fast rules but use the rigor of the trial as a heuristic for choosing what articles to read. Oh, and you can skip the nutritional epidemiology papers (see chapter 9).

For the articles now on your plate, don't read, but actively engage the paper. In your mind, hold on to five questions and dart into the manuscript to find the answers as fast as possible. It's a scavenger hunt for relevant data. Here are a suggested five questions. (1) What was the endpoint improved? Patient centered or surrogate? (2) How big was the magnitude of benefit? Is it clinically relevant? (3) Which patients were included? (4) Was the control arm what I am actually doing in my practice or a straw man? And (5) was crossover used or not used appropriately? (See chapter 9.)

For articles that answer all these questions correctly—a drug improved an important patient-centered endpoint; the benefit was clinically meaningful; the control arm was appropriate; the patients were representative; crossover was used or not used correctly—those are the ones I take for a deep dive.

A deep dive means reading the full paper, reading the supplement, and if the drug receives FDA approval, I start by reading section 14 of the drug label,* which details efficacy studies. For some drugs I am very interested in, I read more of the FDA documentation, such as the medical review, on the same website. As you read, you may hear the voice of the medical writer (see chapter 7) hyping a marginal benefit or a subgroup. Be able to recognize discussion or spin that goes beyond the shown results. With a little practice, it becomes easy.

In case you are wondering how you will have time for all this, I will have to admit that very few trials will make it so far. In my experience, it is just a tiny fraction of papers that make it to my deep dive stage. Maybe one a week, at most, and I follow many journals. At the same time, I want to say that you have to do this. You have to get into the practice of reading these articles fully, of reading supplements. This is the job of the twenty-first-century practitioner. As we have seen in this book, we cannot rely upon the FDA or the guidelines or other professional bodies to deliver the highest-quality, impartial assessment of drugs and trials. We have to do it ourselves. We have to become continual learners. So, congratulations on your degree, now you can start to really study hard—there is simply no other way.

Participate in the Discussion

I started by saying that you should try to keep up with the literature in real time, as articles come out. Why? Because I think it is important

---

* Available at https://www.accessdata.fda.gov/scripts/cder/daf/.

that you join, or at least witness, the conversation. Over the last five years, I have noticed a growing community of health care professionals on Twitter. They are on all social media platforms, to some extent, but in my mind, Twitter has jumped out as the place of the greatest interaction.

In the hours and days after the paper is published, you will see, if you follow like-minded professionals, debate and discourse on the topic. How are others assimilating and interpreting the information? Who is defending and arguing for the results? Who is poking holes in the methods? You want to watch this discussion. I learn things by doing so. And, insofar as you feel comfortable and able, toss out your thoughts. Don't be afraid to be wrong, because most users will not notice if someone else corrects you. Our own missteps are often magnified in our minds but insignificant to others. Only by trial and error do we get better at reading papers.

Listen to Topical Podcasts

It isn't just Twitter or other social media sites where you can learn. There are a number of high-quality podcasts that try to discuss breaking results. I am the host of one called *Plenary Session* (free on Soundcloud, Spotify, and the iTunes store), and the big oncology journals all have a podcast. In all honesty, I struggle with some of the major journals' forays into podcasting—the episodes are often awful—poor audio quality (via phone), unprepared speakers, and so on. If you are a journal editor and want to improve your podcast, call me. I have some tips. But trainees can gain a lot on their daily commute from having a few good medicine podcasts to listen to.

Avoid Financial Conflicts

Besides keeping up with the literature and data on your terms, the other major piece of advice I can offer is to assiduously avoid financial conflicts of interest. I hope to have made the case (in chapters 6 and 7) that these so often distort the interpretation of cancer results. More-

over, many of the problems outlined in chapter 10—our shifting interpretation of commonsense cancer principles—are likely influenced by
these conflicts. In my opinion, although financial conflicts can be quite
large, the industry is still purchasing your attention or loyalty at a low
rate. Your impartiality is worth far more than any gift or consulting
payment, and you should strive to avoid personal financial relationships with for-profit entities in the health care space (aside from your
principal employer).

Be Better Every Day

Many years ago, I was working with a senior oncologist. He had a
patient that afternoon to whom he had to deliver bad news. Despite his
best efforts and multiple lines of therapy, the cancer had steadily gotten worse on scans, and he was going to recommend hospice care. I
had been working with this physician for months and was a fly on the
wall when he went to see the patient.

From my point of view, I witnessed one of those human interactions
that reminds me of what a privilege it is to be a physician. We become
so close to so many people in their most vulnerable times. This senior
oncologist delivered the news better than I could even imagine. He was
clear and kind, warm and regretful. The doctor and patient had known
each other for many years, and it was evident that they cared deeply
about each other. I admit to blinking away tears. At the end of the
conversation, they hugged. It was a warm embrace.

Afterward, I told the senior physician that I thought he did a wonderful job, as well as possible, under the circumstances. He looked
up at me and said he didn't feel that way. "After doing this for 30
years, I can't say that I'm good at it. But I try to be a little bit better
each year."

And, of course, that is why he was so good. Because in his own
mind, he aspired to be a little bit better each year. We should extend
that attitude to everything we do, from our bedside manner, to how we
read the literature, to our thinking, to how we debate and write. Try
to be a bit better each year, and never rest on past accomplishments.

Closing Thoughts

This is a book about cancer health policy. It isn't about the biology of cancer that largely remains untamed, but about human decisions around cancer that are under our control. I hope to have outlined my own thinking on this topic, explaining why I think the magnetic pull of profit, regulatory capture, and hype have resulted in policies that lead us astray from the best interests of people with cancer. Much of that pull is subtle, hard to see, and easy to miss or to ignore.

In part I of this book, I showed how the price of cancer drugs is reaching unsustainable and cruel heights, while the benefits these drugs offer are often marginal or unclear. Part of that obfuscation is due to the rampant use of surrogate endpoints—stand-ins for what matter. But like an old action movie where you notice the stunt double, here, too, the surrogates may fall short. They are often not validated or they poorly capture the effect drugs have on survival or quality of life. Much of their use appears to directly contradict standards voiced by the FDA. Finally, I showed that drug prices are not explained by R&D outlays or how well drugs work; instead, they are merely the by-product of a dysfunctional market that exerts little to no downward pressure.

In part II, I explored the social and political forces behind cancer medicine. Hype is rampant and often paired with spin. Financial conflict pervades. And, we move from fad to fad in cancer medicine—currently we are on the whole genome-sequencing bandwagon. These domains are also the product of a misalignment in policy between what patients need and what special interests desire.

In part III, I tried to teach the intricacies of clinical trials and evidence. What are the principles of oncology that were once common sense, but now increasingly forgotten? How do trials continue to carve out market share but fail to deliver information patients and physicians deserve? Finally, I surveyed the global landscape. The crushing cost of drugs and inappropriate clinical trials agenda has repercussions far beyond the United States.

In part IV, I sought solutions. What can the FDA, the CMS, patients, trainees, and all of us do to push for a better, fairer, more rational system? How should cancer drugs be developed? Who should run trials? How can more impartiality and rigor be added to shift trials back to patients? John Ioannidis, a physician and leading thinker, wrote a paper in 2017 called "Evidence-Based Medicine Has Been Hijacked,"[1] in which he alludes to some of the problems discussed in this book. How do we have more randomized trials than ever, but so much evidence seems a self-fulfilling prophecy—like the non-inferiority trials in chapter 11? My solutions explain how we can commandeer the ship, ways we can steer it back to shore.

When you set out to write a book it seems a daunting and insurmountable task, but when you finish you wish you could add so much more. My colleagues and I have a number of ongoing research projects on many of the themes of this book, and I wish I could share our emerging findings, but I based this book on data that had already been published.

Conclusion

Oncology, when practiced well, is both science and art. We are able to cure disease or to restore function for many patients, helping them live a long and good life. There are many others for whom we can temporarily improve symptoms or survival, and there are some for whom we provide, at best, human comfort. We cannot forget that despite the talk of miracles and game changers and revolutions and cures, cancer still robs too many years from too many people. We must do better. Some of the challenges of biology may take decades, centuries, or even millennia to fully crack, but in the meantime, the policies and funding and evidence that remain under our control should be optimized to always and only pursue what's best for patients. Now is the time to start.

Epilogue
The Hallmarks of Successful Cancer Policy

Dividing things where the natural joints are, and not trying to break any part,
after the manner of a bad carver
PLATO, *PHAEDRUS*

A S IS often the case in life, it was right before this book went to the printers that I realized one way I might have said things better. In my case, however, it is not too late for a last thought. The problems we encountered span broad domains: conflicts of interest, endpoints that do not measure what matters, difficulty applying trial results to average people with cancer, lofty and unsustainable prices, suboptimal research funding, and duplicative, redundant, uninformative, and even unethical trials. Yet, perhaps the complexity of cancer policy can be distilled to six essential opportunities—six domains where we might realign the incentives in the system to serve people with cancer. I propose the six hallmarks of successful cancer policy are *independence, evidence, relevance, affordability, possibility,* and *agenda.* Allow me to show how consideration of these six categories could lead to more fruitful cancer research and practice.

Independence—Entities Must Be Free to Advocate for Their Constituencies

The first principle of successful cancer policy is independence. It is important for the distinct parties in cancer medicine to be able to advocate for their constituencies free from the influence of others. Inde-

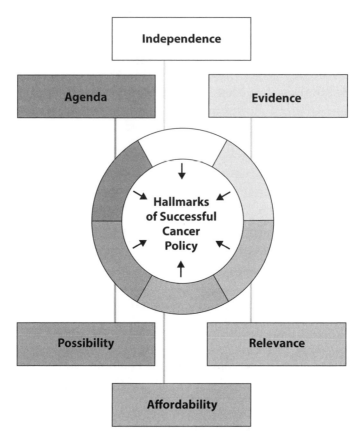

Figure E.1. Hallmarks of successful cancer policy

pendence is a hallmark of fair and just systems, including the separate and coequal branches of US government as well as the parties that interact in just judicial systems (the judge is not paid by the prosecution). Unfortunately, we have seen a threat to cancer medicine's independence through the volume and scope of payments from the biopharmaceutical industry (chapters 6 and 7). These payments disincentivize criticism of the industry and favor the use of marginal products based on inadequate evidence.

Independence would untangle many of these dueling roles. Patient groups should feel comfortable criticizing the high and unsustainable price of drugs. Academics must be able to serve as impartial arbiters of medical evidence, particularly when that evidence is gray, as is often the case in cancer medicine.[1] Guideline writers can draw upon their clinical experience but may operate best by avoiding potential conflicts of interest.

Independence that exists in other policy spaces, such as courtrooms, must be expanded to cancer medicine. It should be clear that independence does not imply silos or no communication among constituencies. Groups that frequently interact can do so in the absence of financial payments. Again, the analogy of the courtroom is relevant. Prosecutors, defense attorneys, and judges often convene to engage in a process that strives for fair and just decisions, yet at no point are there financial ties among these three parties. The presence of such ties would be problematic and, in many cases, would violate the law.

Evidence—Measure What Matters, and Do It Fairly

The second hallmark of a successful cancer policy is the generation of high-quality evidence. Evidence refers to the need to conduct trials that ask whether tests and treatments improve outcomes that matter: overall survival and quality of life.

Reliable evidence extends beyond endpoints. Studies must be well-done randomized controlled trials without tipping the scale. This means (1) using non-inferiority trials only when the design makes sense, for example, when the new drug is cheaper, less toxic, or more convenient than the old drug;[2,3] (2) making sure changes in dose due to side effects are fair and balanced;[4] (3) comparing a new drug to the best standard of care; [5] and (4) using crossover correctly: never in a trial that asks if a drug works for the very first time but always in a trial that hopes to move a successful drug earlier in treatment.

Relevance—Our Studies Must Aid Average People with Cancer

Relevance is related to evidence but focuses on whether results are useful to the average person with cancer. As we have seen, cancer trials recruit the young and otherwise healthy, and a drug with marginal benefits and toxicity in this group may find its benefits erode when given to older and frailer people. To achieve relevance, cancer clinical trials must ask questions in broad populations without irrational restrictions.

When it comes to evidence and relevance, the temptation to cheat is too great if the designers of a study have their career or billions of dollars at stake. We need nonconflicted groups to design and conduct these studies (detailed in chapter 14).

Affordability—Successful Therapies Must Be Broadly Available

It is imperative that drugs are affordable for this simple reason: an unaffordable drug is no better than no drug at all. There are a number of proposed solutions to lower cancer drug prices. Many are technical and dry, and I refer interested readers to this review on the topic for specific ideas.[6]

One under-recognized aspect of affordability is the importance of separating health care and research. Practices found in health care have shown they offer benefits, while practices under investigation refer to treatments that are promising but still uncertain. Societies pay for health care and research in different ways and different amounts. Health care is paid for through a combination of governments, insurance companies, and out-of-pocket expenses. Research is funded through public research dollars, biopharmaceutical companies, and nongovernmental foundations. The amount of money spent for each of these varies substantially. For instance, in the United States, national health care expenditure totals $3.5 trillion, or roughly $10,000 per person,[7] while the total research budget is approximately $110 billion, or $300 per person (the pharma R&D budget is $71 billion[8] and the National Institutes of Health is $39.2 billion).[9] In other words, our research budget is roughly 3% of our health care budget.

What exactly is the correct ratio of spending on research versus care remains an unresolved question,* but it is important to separate the two for the simple reason that societies may choose to prioritize these ex-

* Over the course of this book, I have argued for more research funding, particularly to test unproven medicine.

penditures differently. Yet, increasingly, we have seen the lines blur and research investigations utilize health care mechanisms for payment. This results in inefficient, costly, and uncertain health care spending, and it is unsustainable.

Consider the push to sequence the tumor of every person with cancer (chapter 8). This is still unproven, but many have lobbied for insurance companies to pay for this service. In 2018, the CMS agreed to provide coverage of Foundation Medicine's F1CDx for all advanced or metastatic solid tumors,[10] effectively shifting the cost of such sequencing to health care budgets.[11] Some research papers using broad sequencing and paired therapy admit to having insurance providers pay for the off-label anticancer medications,[12,13] further transferring the cost.

The challenge with this shift—moving unproven interventions from research to health care—is that the costs escalate tremendously, and the information collected from such efforts may be minimal. For instance, the CMS removed a requirement to track outcomes for patients being treated with off-label drugs after an F1Cdx assay in the final decision,[14] which limits the ability for patients, physicians, and policy makers to judge the success or failure of this costly coverage decision.

Successful health care policy must balance, realign, and optimize the ratio of spending on care and research. We must be cautious not to fund uncertain interventions through mechanisms meant for payment of proven therapies. While we may need to spend more on research, the wrong way to achieve that is to falsely declare that an uncertain intervention works. Such a system is inefficient, exposing far more people to investigational interventions than would be necessary in a clinical trial. Ultimately, this would incur greater expenditure and may not even answer whether the practice works as intended.

Possibility—The Preclinical Pipeline Must Be Expanded

The fifth hallmark of successful cancer policy is possibility. Possibility refers to the development of a big cancer treatment pipeline. The need for a big pipeline is illustrated by the simple fact that it is difficult, if not impossible, to predict what cancer treatments will work. Contopoulos-

Ioannidis and colleagues found that just a tiny fraction (5/101) of highly promising basic science findings made it to the clinic decades later,[15] and in cancer medicine, it is often serendipitous or unexpected findings that deliver. A recent article profiling Nobel laureate James Allison states that he was called "foolish" for trying to pursue immune therapy.[16] It is hard to know across the timescale of decades what laboratory findings may result in successful therapies.

For this reason, successful cancer policy must include a wide-bore pipeline with strong, sustained, continuous, reliable, and growing NCI funding for preclinical science. This should be done broadly and avoid the risk of fad funding cycles, as occurred with the enthusiasm for the human genome project and genome-driven cancer medicine.[17,18] Possibility also means allocating a sizable proportion of NIH funding to blue skies science, defined as science done merely to understand the world and not focused on delivering (unrealistic) promises of imminent translation.

One of the major challenges is the inefficiency with which funds are dispersed. Fang and colleagues found that NIH peer review percentile scores, which determine whether grants are funded or not, have nearly no correlation with metrics of research productivity, such as citation scores.[19] Among grants with percentile scores of 20 or better (the range in which funding decisions are typically made), receiving a higher score is akin to a coin flip in choosing the project destined to produce greater citations. This phenomenon is not unique to the United States but affects all nations. Analyses from Australia, France, and Canada found problems with research funding.[20,21]

There have been a number of proposals to fix the current system. These include: funding scientists based on prior publications and a one-page proposal,[22] polling other scientists,[23] funding all proposals with less funding,[24] or a modified lottery,[25] whereby proposals that meet a basic cutoff of soundness are randomly selected. All of these proposals can be tested the same way we would test a drug or surgery.[24] Here is one such randomized trial (fig. E.2).

Endpoints can include measures of research productivity, translation, and equitable and just funding.

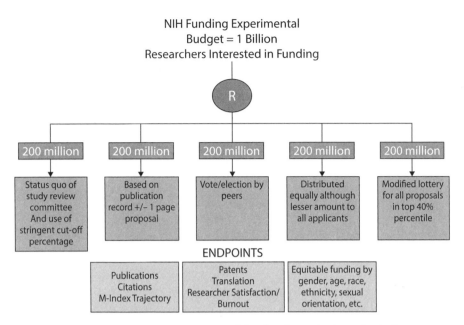

Figure E.2. A proposed randomized trial for deciding which method of research funding is optimal. In this hypothetical a billion dollars of funding is equally allocated to four intervention and one control arm, and a diverse set of endpoints are assessed.

Agenda—The Overall Cancer Trials Landscape Must Maximize the Contribution of Participants

The current cancer clinical trials research agenda, or the set of all clinical trials, is not often discussed, but it is vitally important. As we saw in chapter 9, the way you think about one drug, bevacizumab, depends on whether you view every separate trial as an island unto itself, or consider it alongside the fact that the drug has been tested in so many different trials. By chance alone, some of these may be positive. When we adjusted for this fact, many of the trials lost their statistical significance.[26]

It is important to minimize bias in specific cancer studies, but deciding what questions to ask, in what order, and with what resources is also vulnerable to bias. We need a formal system that is capable of asking the best questions in the best order for people with cancer. The most direct solution is to create and fund a large, nonconflicted clinical-trials portfolio at the multinational, governmental level (chapter 14). Such a group can work to improve the relevance and evidence of trials, as discussed before, but also help decide which questions should be prioritized.

Cancer research cannot be both duplicative and absent. We have to strike the right balance. People with cancer are the scarcest and most precious part of cancer clinical trials, and thinking broadly about the overarching trials agenda, its efficiency and harm to participants is the final hallmark of successful cancer policy. It is a way to honor their contributions.

Conclusion

The challenges in cancer policy discussed in this book have been diverse, but I believe these six fundamental arenas of reform could lead to realignment of incentives with the best interests of people with cancer. These hallmarks are: striving for *independence* among actors in the cancer drug space, generating *evidence* that is reliable, conducting trials that are *relevant* for practicing clinicians in the real world, creating therapies that are *affordable* and available globally, enlarging the *promise* of the preclinical pipeline, and, finally, developing a large nonconflicted clinical-trials *agenda* to sort out which interventions work and which do not. These concepts are often intertwined, and durable reform of cancer policy may need to address all domains. I hope this book may help guide future research and thinking on this topic.

accelerated approval. A type of drug approval granted by the US Food and Drug Administration on the basis of surrogate endpoints thought reasonably likely to predict clinical benefit. Accelerated approval typically required further postmarket studies to confirm efficacy.

adjuvant therapy. Any therapy used to treat patients after their primary treatment to increase its effectiveness

all-cause mortality. Death for any reason

American Society of Clinical Oncology (ASCO). A professional society of oncologists

American Society of Hematology (ASH). A professional society of hematologists

ASCO. *See* American Society of Clinical Oncology

autologous bone marrow transplant. An intensive therapy where stem cells are collected, a lethal dose of chemotherapy is administered, and the stem cells returned to rescue the patient

bioplausible. Refers to interventions that make biologic sense that they should work but remain unproven

CAR-T therapy (Chimeric antigen receptor T-Cell therapy). A cancer treatment where the body's own T-cells are removed, inserted with a genetic instruction to target a particular cancer protein, and given to the patient through a vein

checkpoint inhibitors. A class of anticancer drugs that work by unleashing the immune system against the cancer cell, a form of immunotherapy

chemoprevention. A drug or therapy given to prevent cancer

chemotherapy. A broad category of cancer drugs, though colloquially refers to cytotoxic drugs

clinical endpoint. An endpoint that intrinsically matters to patients, such as living longer or better; contrast against surrogate endpoint

clinical trial. A formal study of a cancer interventions

comparative effectiveness. A comparison between two effective treatments

composite endpoint. An endpoint of a trial where one of several events or occurrences may count toward reaching the endpoint; for example, progression-free survival

conflict of interest. A competing or dueling duty or obligation. Typically a payment from the pharmaceutical industry to a physician.

consolidation therapy. A therapy given after initial cancer treatment, meant to deepen the response, increase the durability of the response, or increase the curative fraction

correlation coefficient. A numerical measure of how closely two variables are linked

crossover. The characteristic in cancer trials where patients initially allocated to the control or placebo arm are later given access to the investigational agent

CT scan. A computed tomography scan, a highly detailed image

cytotoxic drugs. Chemotherapy agents that preferentially kill cells undergoing division. Their side effects often target hair, gastrointestinal tracts, and bone marrow because these cells divide more rapidly than other healthy cells. Chemotherapy alone can cure several cancers—testicular and lymphoma, for instance—and increase cure rates after surgery for many others—lung, breast, and colon, for example.

DCIS (ductal carcinoma in situ). A premalignant lesion in breast cancer that is the subject of constant debate regarding its significance

disease-free survival (DFS). The time until cancer recurs or a person dies, whichever comes first. A composite, time-to-event, endpoint.

effect size. The magnitude of benefit or harm

EMA (European Medicines Agency). The European analog to the US FDA

epidemiological studies. Studies investigating the distribution of a disease or condition within populations

exclusion criteria. A list of criteria that determine a person would not be eligible for a clinical study

genome sequencing. Identifying the order of the DNA bases in the cancer cell

hazard ratio. A dimensionless measure comparing the ratio of the rate of events in one arm against another; in and of itself a hazard ratio is impossible to interpret with patients.

hematopoietic cells. Cells that form into the blood, platelets, and infection-fighting white cells

historically controlled trials. Studies where the outcomes for consecutively treated patients in one period of time are compared against those from a prior period; a type of study known for frequently exaggerating the benefit of therapies

immunotherapy. Immunotherapy drugs are those that utilize the body's immune system to attack cancer. There are several classes: (1) Cancer therapeutic vaccines are vaccines given to people who already have cancer to encourage their own body to attack the tumor. (2) Cancer checkpoint inhibitors are a blockbuster class of medications that make it more difficult for cancer to escape the body's immune system, and they are often described as "unleashing" the immune system. (3) Cellular therapies are made outside of the body and re-infused in order to attack cancer. The most notable version in recent years is called CAR-T. (4) Finally, bone marrow transplants from one person to another, which have existed for decades, are a form of immunotherapy.

inclusion criteria. The set of requirements a person must fulfill in order to enter a study

indication (drug indication). The specific cancer, setting (adjuvant vs. metastatic), line of therapy (first, second, etc.), and other requirements to receive a therapy. Drugs are approved for specific indications.

Indolent biology. Refers to a cancer that naturally grows slower than average

JAMA. (*Journal of the American Medical Association*). A prestigious medical journal

LDL. Low-density lipoprotein

line of therapy. The first, second, third, etc. course of therapy prescribed for metastatic cancer

maintenance therapy. A drug given indefinitely or for a prolonged period of time after a fixed course of therapy

malignant. Cancer or cancerous

meta-analysis. An analytic method that allows one to pool the results of many studies together

metastatic. Having spread beyond the initial site of cancer, for instance, when breast cancer spreads to the liver

monoclonal antibody. A class of drugs that are large antibodies, or immune molecules that are usually exquisitely targeted against cell surface markers

MRI. Magnetic resonance imaging

National Cancer Institute. The US federal agency in charge of cancer research, a part of the NIH

National Institutes of Health (NIH). The major federal research funder for science

NEJM (*New England Journal of Medicine*). A prestigious medical journal

non-inferior. A form of statistical comparison that asks if one treatment is no worse than a predefined margin or delta than another

observational studies. Studies that observe the outcomes or characteristics of patients who receive treatments as recommended by their physicians

ODAC (Oncology Drug Advisory Committee). A governmental panel that advises the FDA as to whether the harm-benefit balance of a novel drug approval or indication is favorable

off-label use. Using a drug for a purpose not explicitly granted by the FDA

overall survival. The percent of or number of people alive. Typically overall survival and all cause mortality are opposites of each other, and add up to 100%.

palliative treatment. Treatment that improves symptoms, or extends life, but does not result in cures

PFS. *See* progression-free survival

pharma. The pharmaceutical industry, or drug companies

phase 1 study. A type of experimental trial that seeks to identify a safe dose of a new cancer medication or combination to take forward in phase 2

phase 2 study. A trial that seeks to determine if a drug has promise or activity in a particular cancer setting

phase 3 studies. A large clinical study, typically randomized, that asks whether a drug improves outcomes beyond or in addition to standard of care

plenary session. The most important session of a large conference; also the name of a popular and exciting podcast

post-protocol therapy. Treatments given after therapies on a clinical trial (on-protocol therapies)

precision oncology. A popular topic in cancer medicine, for which the definition has shifted (see chapter 8) but typically involves the use of genomics to prescribe drugs to people with cancer

primary endpoint. The primary outcome that is investigated in a study. Most studies are designed and suited only to make firm conclusions regarding the primary endpoint.

progression (tumor progression, cancer progression). Defined in chapters 2 and 3; Progression typically occurs when tumors grow more than 20% from their smallest size, or there are new tumors on imaging.

progression-free survival. The time until either progression or death, whichever comes first. Also a composite endpoint and a time-to-event endpoint.

propensity score. A technique that attempts to isolate the effect of an intervention by accounting for factors that affect the likelihood of getting that intervention

p-value. The probability one would have observed this result or a more extreme result if the null hypothesis (that there is no difference between the experimental and control arms) is true

quality adjusted life-year (QALY). One year of healthy living, which is discounted for states of being sick or infirm

R&D. Research and development

randomized controlled trial (RCT). A clinical experiment where participants are randomly assigned to one treatment or another and their outcomes compared. The best way to ascertain the efficacy of a cancer therapy, performed for interventions that are thought to be of benefit, with modest or marginal effect size. For this reason, it applies to nearly all biomedical interventions.

recurrence (local, distant). The reoccurrence of a cancer that was treated with curative intent

refractory. A cancer that has grown while receiving therapies or after receiving some therapy

retrospective studies. Observational studies that are conducted looking backward. For instance, we ask a question in 2018, but look at patients from 2005 to 2010 to answer it.

RR (Response rate). The percentage of patients experiencing tumor response

RO1 Funding. A major grant most researchers hope to get from the National Institutes of Health

secondary endpoint. An endpoint also of interest in a cancer trial, but not the primary endpoint, for which the trial may not be suited to render a firm verdict

single agent activity. The percentage of patients who experience response from one drug administered all by itself

single-arm trial. An experimental trial of a cancer therapy where all patients receive the treatment, and there is no comparison group

solid cancers / solid tumors. A common distinction in oncology is made between tumors of the solid organs and those of the hematopoietic system (blood cancers or hematologic malignancies).

Stage of cancer. Cancer is staged the first time it is diagnosed, often as stage 1, 2, 3, or 4, with higher numbers typically carrying a worse prognosis.

statistically significant. Having a p-value less than a predefined cutoff, typically lower than 0.05

stem cells. Cells that can grow or develop into normal cells or tissues

super responder. A patient who experiences a dramatic response to an anti-cancer drug

surrogate endpoint. A surrogate endpoint is an intermediary or stand-in endpoint. It is meant to represent a clinical or patient-centered endpoint, such as living longer or having an improved quality of life, but can be measured sooner or more easily. Clinical endpoints are ones that inherently matter to patients, and surrogates are those that merely approximate clinical endpoints.

surrogate validation study. A type of analysis that asks whether a surrogate endpoint reliably predicts which agents will go on to improve survival or quality of life

targeted drugs. Small molecules and antibodies (recall chapter 1) that are directed against specific cancer proteins or molecules

time-to-event endpoints. Endpoints that occur only after time has elapsed from the start of a study

time-to-progression. Similar to PFS, but death is not treated as an endpoint; instead it's a reason to censor the analysis.

tumor response. If cancer shrinks more than an arbitrary threshold, typically 30% from the starting size, as assessed on imaging

US Food and Drug Association (FDA). The regulatory agency in charge of approving what drugs come to the US market, and what additional uses they may be marketed for.

REFERENCES

Introduction

1. Bailar JC, Smith EM. Progress against Cancer? *New Engl J Med.* 1986; 314(19):1226–1232.

2. Kolata G. Breast cancer: anguish, mystery and hope. *New York Times Magazine.* April 24, 1988: 6006042. https://www.nytimes.com/1988/04/24 /magazine/breat-cancer-anguish-mystery-and-hope.html. Accessed August 2, 2019.

3. Antman K, Gale R. Advanced breast cancer: high-dose chemotherapy and bone marrow autotransplants. *Ann Intern Med.* 1988;108(4):570–574.

4. Eddy DM. High-dose chemotherapy with autologous bone marrow transplantation for the treatment of metastatic breast cancer. *J Clin Oncol.* 1992;10(4): 657–670.

5. Leff L. MD. Mother's chance at life hinges on trial. *Washington Post.* April 17, 1990.

6. Mahaney FX, Jr. Bone marrow transplants used against advanced breast cancer. *J Natl Cancer Ins.* 1989;81(18):1352–1353.

7. Kolata G. Women resist trials to test marrow transplants. *New York Times.* February 15, 1995.

8. Hillner BE, Smith TJ, Desch CE. Efficacy and cost-effectiveness of autologous bone marrow transplantation in metastatic breast cancer: estimates using decision analysis while awaiting clinical trial results. *JAMA.* 1992;267(15): 2055–2061.

9. Kolata G, Eichenwald K. HOPE FOR SALE: a special report.; business thrives on unproven care, leaving science behind. *New York Times.* October 3, 1999.

10. Bezwoda WR, Seymour L, Dansey RD. High-dose chemotherapy with hematopoietic rescue as primary treatment for metastatic breast cancer: a randomized trial. *J Clin Oncol.* 1995;13(10):2483–2489.

11. Lippman ME. High-dose chemotherapy plus autologous bone marrow transplantation for metastatic breast cancer. *New Engl J Med.* 2000;342(15): 1119–1120.

12. Hayes DF. Book Review. *New Engl J Med.* 2007;357(10):1059–1060.

13. Mello MM, Brennan TA. The controversy over high-dose chemotherapy with autologous bone marrow transplant for breast cancer. *Health Affairs.* 2001;20(5):101–117.

Chapter 1. The Basics of Cancer Drugs

1. Druker BJ, Talpaz M, Resta DJ, et al. Efficacy and safety of a specific inhibitor of the BCR-ABL tyrosine kinase in chronic myeloid leukemia. *New Engl J Med.* 2001;344(14):1031–1037. doi: 10.1056/nejm200104053441401.

2. Bower H, Bjorkholm M, Dickman PW, et al. Life expectancy of patients with chronic myeloid leukemia approaches the life expectancy of the general population. *J Clin Oncol* 2016;34(24):2851–2857. doi: 10.1200/jco.2015.66.2866 [published Online First: 2016/06/22].

3. Fojo T, Mailankody S, Lo A. Unintended consequences of expensive cancer therapeutics—the pursuit of marginal indications and a me-too mentality that stifles innovation and creativity: the John Conley lecture. *JAMA Otolaryngol.* 2014;140(12):1225–1236. doi: 10.1001/jamaoto.2014.1570.

4. Salas-Vega S, Iliopoulos O, Mossialos E. Assessment of overall survival, quality of life, and safety benefits associated with new cancer medicines. *JAMA Oncol* 2017;3(3):382–390. doi: 10.1001/jamaoncol.2016.4166.

5. Hurwitz H, Fehrenbacher L, Novotny W, et al. Bevacizumab plus irinotecan, fluorouracil, and leucovorin for metastatic colorectal cancer. *New Engl J Med.* 2004;350(23):2335–2342. doi: 10.1056/NEJMoa032691.

6. Prasad V. Overestimating the benefit of cancer drugs. *JAMA Oncol.* 2017. doi: 10.1001/jamaoncol.2017.0107.

7. FDA Approval for Sorafenib Tosylate. November 26. National Cancer Institute, 2013.

8. Llovet JM, Ricci S, Mazzaferro V, et al. Sorafenib in advanced hepatocellular carcinoma. *New Engl J Med.* 2008;359(4):378–390. doi: 10.1056/NEJMoa0708857.

9. Sanoff HK, Chang Y, Lund JL, et al. Sorafenib effectiveness in advanced hepatocellular carcinoma. *Oncologist.* 2016;21(9):1113–1120. doi: 10.1634/theoncologist.2015-0478 [published Online First: 2016/05/18].

10. Scher KS, Hurria A. Under-representation of older adults in cancer registration trials: known problem, little progress. *J Clin Oncol.* 2012;30(17):2036–2038. doi: 10.1200/JCO.2012.41.6727.

11. Sekeres MA. Strict clinical trial eligibility criteria exclude patients most likely to benefit from cancer treatment. *HemOnc Today.* February 8, 2017. https://www.healio.com/hematology-oncology/myeloma/news/online/%7Bc9859d83-a776-40b5-ba20-fc31f3d283ed%7D/strict-clinical-trial-eligibility-criteria-exclude-patients-most-likely-to-benefit-from-cancer-treatment. Accessed August 2, 2019.

12. Fehrenbacher L, Ackerson L, Somkin C. Randomized clinical trial eligibility rates for chemotherapy (CT) and antiangiogenic therapy (AAT) in a population-based cohort of newly diagnosed non-small cell lung cancer (NSCLC) patients. *J Clin Oncol.* 2009;27(15_suppl):6538–6538. doi: 10.1200/jco.2009.27.15_suppl.6538.

13. Mailankody S, Prasad V. Overall survival in cancer drug trials as a new surrogate end point for overall survival in the real world. *JAMA Oncol.* 2017;3(7):889–890. doi: 10.1001/jamaoncol.2016.5296 [published Online First: 2016/11/29].

14. Tannock IF, Amir E, Booth CM, et al. Relevance of randomised controlled

trials in oncology. *Lancet Oncol.* 2016;17(12):e560–e567. doi: 10.1016/s1470-2045(16)30572-1 [published Online First: 2016/12/08].

15. Booth CM, Cescon DW, Wang L, et al. Evolution of the randomized controlled trial in oncology over three decades. *J Clin Oncol.* 2008;26(33):5458–5464. doi: 10.1200/jco.2008.16.5456 [published Online First: 2008/10/29].

16. Seruga B, Hertz PC, Wang L, et al. Absolute benefits of medical therapies in phase III clinical trials for breast and colorectal cancer. *Ann Oncol.* 2010;21(7): 1411–8. doi: 10.1093/annonc/mdp552 [published Online First: 2009/12/03].

17. Sacher AG, Le LW, Leighl NB. Shifting patterns in the interpretation of phase III clinical trial outcomes in advanced non-small-cell lung cancer: the bar is dropping. *J Clin Oncol* 2014;32(14):1407–1411. doi: 10.1200/jco.2013.52.7804 [published Online First: 2014/03/05].

18. Mailankody S, Prasad V. Five years of cancer drug approvals: innovation, efficacy, and costs. *JAMA Oncol.* 2015;1(4):539–540. doi: 10.1001/jamaoncol .2015.0373.

19. Fox M. Global cancer drug market grows to $107 billion. NBC News2016. Updated June 2, 2016. Available from: https://www.nbcnews.com/health/cancer /global-cancer-drug-market-grows-107-billion-n584481. Accessed October 5, 2017.

20. Silverman E. Sharp rise in cancer drug spending forecast, but access remains a problem. STAT. https://www.statnews.com/pharmalot/2016/06/02/spending -cancer-drugs-forecast-access-still-problem/. Updated June 2, 2016. Accessed October 5, 2017.

21. Bach PB. Limits on Medicare's ability to control rising spending on cancer drugs. *New Engl J Med.* 2009;360(6):626–633. doi: 10.1056/NEJMhpr0807774.

22. Dusetzina SB. Drug pricing trends for orally administered anticancer medications reimbursed by commercial health plans, 2000–2014. *JAMA Oncol.* 2016;2(7):960–961. doi: 10.1001/jamaoncol.2016.0648.

23. Neumann PJ, Cohen JT, Weinstein MC. Updating cost-effectiveness—the curious resilience of the $50,000-per-QALY threshold. *New Engl J Med.* 2014; 371(9):796–797. doi: 10.1056/NEJMp1405158.

24. Goldstein DA. The ethical and practical challenges of value-based cancer care at the patient's bedside. *JAMA Oncol.* 2016;2(7):860–861. doi: 10.1001 /jamaoncol.2016.0535.

25. Goldstein DA, Ahmad BB, Chen Q, et al. Cost-effectiveness analysis of regorafenib for metastatic colorectal cancer. *J Clin Oncol* 2015;33(32):3727–3732. doi: 10.1200/jco.2015.61.9569 [published Online First: 2015/08/26].

26. Durkee BY, Qian Y, Pollom EL, et al. Cost-effectiveness of pertuzumab in human epidermal growth factor receptor 2–positive metastatic breast cancer. *J Clin Oncol.* 2016;34(9):902–909. doi: 10.1200/jco.2015.62.9105 [published Online First: 2015/09/10].

27. Goldstein DA, Chen Q, Ayer T, et al. First- and second-line bevacizumab in addition to chemotherapy for metastatic colorectal cancer: a United States–based cost-effectiveness analysis. *J Clin Oncol.* 2015;33(10):1112–1118. doi: 10.1200 /jco.2014.58.4904 [published Online First: 2015/02/19].

28. Hill A, Gotham D, Fortunak J, et al. Target prices for mass production of tyrosine kinase inhibitors for global cancer treatment. *BMJ Open.* 2016;6(1). doi: 10.1136/bmjopen-2015-009586.

29. Kelley B. Industrialization of mAb production technology: the bioprocessing industry at a crossroads. *mAbs* 2009;1(5):443–452.

30. Avorn J. The $2.6 billion pill—methodologic and policy considerations. *New Engl J Med.* 2015;372(20):1877–1879. doi: 10.1056/NEJMp1500848.

31. Young B SM. Rx R&D Myths: The Case against the Drug Industry's R&D "Scare Card." Washington, DC: Public Citizen's Congress Watch, 2001.

Chapter 2. Surrogate Endpoints in Cancer

1. Moertel CG, Hanley JA. The effect of measuring error on the results of therapeutic trials in advanced cancer. *Cancer.* 1976;Jul;38(1):388–94. https://www.ncbi.nlm.nih.gov/pubmed/947531.

2. Eisenhauer EA, Therasse P, Bogaerts J, et al. New response evaluation criteria in solid tumours: Revised RECIST guideline (version 1.1). *Eur J Cancer.* 2009;45(2):228–247. doi: https://doi.org/10.1016/j.ejca.2008.10.026.

3. Dhingra K. Rociletinib: has the TIGER lost a few of its stripes? *Ann Oncol.* 2016;27(6):1161–1164. doi: 10.1093/annonc/mdw140 [published Online First: 2016/04/06].

4. Schiavon G, Ruggiero A, Schoffski P, et al. Tumor volume as an alternative response measurement for imatinib treated GIST patients. *PLoS One.* 2012;7(11): e48372. doi: 10.1371/journal.pone.0048372 [published Online First: 2012/11/08].

5. Kim C, Prasad V. Strength of validation for surrogate end points used in the US Food and Drug Administration's approval of oncology drugs. *Mayo Clin Proc.* 2016;91(6):713–725. doi: 10.1016/j.mayocp.2016.02.012.

6. Kay A, Higgins J, Day AG, et al. Randomized controlled trials in the era of molecular oncology: methodology, biomarkers, and end points. *Ann Oncol.* 2012;23. doi: 10.1093/annonc/mdr492.

7. Miller K, Wang M, Gralow J, et al. Paclitaxel plus bevacizumab versus paclitaxel alone for metastatic breast cancer. *New Engl J Med.* 2007;357(26): 2666–2676. doi: 10.1056/NEJMoa072113.

8. Prasad V, Vandross A. Failing to improve overall survival because postprotocol survival is long: fact, myth, excuse or improper study design? *J Cancer Res Clin.* 2014;140(4):521–524. doi: 10.1007/s00432-014-1590-x [published Online First: 2014/01/30].

9. Carpenter D, Kesselheim AS, Joffe S. Reputation and precedent in the bevacizumab decision. *New Engl J Med.*2011;365. doi: 10.1056/NEJMp1107201.

10. US Food and Drug Administration. Proposed Text of Labeling for the Drug-Annotated Mylotarg™ (gemtuzumab ozogamicin for Injection). https://www.accessdata.fda.gov/drugsatfda_docs/label/2000/21174lbl.pdf. Accessed August 2, 2019.

11. Petersdorf SH, Kopecky KJ, Slovak M, et al. A phase 3 study of gemtuzumab ozogamicin during induction and postconsolidation therapy in younger patients with acute myeloid leukemia. *Blood* 2013;121(24):4854–4860. doi: 10.1182/blood-2013-01-466706.

12. Nelson R. Gemtuzumab voluntarily withdrawn from US market [Online]: Medscape 2010 [updated June 21, 2010. Available from: http://www.medscape.com/viewarticle/723957, accessed September 9, 2018.

13. Validity of surrogate endpoints in oncology. Executive summary of rapid

report A10–05, Version 1.1. Institute for Quality and Efficiency in Health Care: Executive Summaries. Cologne, Germany: Institute for Quality and Efficiency in Health Care (IQWiG) (c) IQWiG (Institute for Quality and Efficiency in Health Care). 2005.

14. Prasad V, Kim C, Burotto M, et al. The strength of association between surrogate end points and survival in oncology: a systematic review of trial-level meta-analyses. *JAMA Intern Med.* 2015;175. doi: 10.1001/jamainternmed.2015.2829.

15. Gyawali B, Hwang T. Prevalence of quality of life (QoL) outcomes and association with survival in cancer clinical trials. 2018 ASCO Annual Meeting Poster Session Health Services Research, Clinical Informatics, and Quality of Care. *J Clin Oncol.* 36, 2018 (suppl;abst 6573), 2018.

16. Kovic B, Jin X, Kennedy S, et al. Evaluating progression-free survival as a surrogate outcome for health-related quality of life in oncology: a systematic review and quantitative analysis. *JAMA Intern Med.* 2018. doi: 10.1001/jamainternmed.2018.4710.

17. Jefferson T, Jones M, Doshi P, et al. Oseltamivir for influenza in adults and children: systematic review of clinical study reports and summary of regulatory comments. *BMJ.* 2014;348. doi: 10.1136/bmj.g2545.

18. Prasad VK, Cifu AS. *Ending Medical Reversal: Improving Outcomes, Saving Lives.* Baltimore: Johns Hopkins University Press, 2015.

19. Chen E, Joshi S, Tran A, et al. Estimation of study time reduction using surrogate end points rather than overall survival in oncology clinical trials. *JAMA Intern Med.* 2019;179(5):642–647. https://jamanetwork.com/journals/jamainternalmedicine/fullarticle/2729389.

20. Kemp R, Prasad V. Surrogate endpoints in oncology: when are they acceptable for regulatory and clinical decisions, and are they currently overused? *BMC Medicine.* 2017;15(1):134. doi: 10.1186/s12916-017-0902-9.

Chapter 3. The Use and Misuse of Surrogate Endpoints for Drug Approvals

1. Kim C, Prasad V. Cancer drugs approved on the basis of a surrogate end point and subsequent overall survival: an analysis of 5 years of US Food and Drug Administration approvals. *JAMA Intern Med.* 2015;175. doi: 10.1001/jamainternmed.2015.5868.

2. Davis C, Naci H, Gurpinar E, et al. Availability of evidence of benefits on overall survival and quality of life of cancer drugs approved by European Medicines Agency: retrospective cohort study of drug approvals 2009–13. *BMJ.* 2017;359. doi: 10.1136/bmj.j4530.

3. Dagher R, Johnson J, Williams G, et al. Accelerated approval of oncology products: a decade of experience. *J Natl Cancer Ins.* 2004;96(20):1500–1509. doi: 10.1093/jnci/djh279 [published Online First: 2004/10/21].

4. Pazdur R. Endpoints for assessing drug activity in clinical trials. *Oncologist* 2008;13. doi: 10.1634/theoncologist.13-S2-19.

5. Kim C, Prasad V. Strength of validation for surrogate end points used in the US Food and Drug Administration's approval of oncology drugs. *Mayo Clin Proc.* 2016;91(6):713–725. doi: https://doi.org/10.1016/j.mayocp.2016.02.012.

6. Blumenthal GM, Karuri SW, Zhang H, et al. Overall response rate, progression-free survival, and overall survival with targeted and standard therapies in advanced non-small-cell lung cancer: US Food and Drug Administration trial-level and patient-level analyses. *J Clin Oncol.* 2015;33(9):1008–1014. doi: 10.1200 /jco.2014.59.0489.

7. Cortazar P, Zhang L, Untch M, et al. Pathological complete response and long-term clinical benefit in breast cancer: the CTNeoBC pooled analysis. *Lancet.* 2014;384. doi: 10.1016/s0140–6736(13)62422–8.

8. Baselga J, Campone M, Piccart M, et al. Everolimus in postmenopausal hormone-receptor-positive advanced breast cancer. *New Engl J Med.* 2012;366. doi: 10.1056/NEJMoa1109653.

9. Gyawali B, Prasad V. Same data; different interpretations. *J Clin Oncol.* 2016;34(31):3729–3732. doi: 10.1200/JCo.2016.68.2021.

10. Fauber J. Slippery slope: a targeted therapy that misses the mark? Afinitor racks up FDA approvals, but where is the evidence? *Medpage Today.* December 13, 2015. https://www.medpagetoday.com/special-reports/slipperyslope/55170. Accessed October 17, 2017.

11. Woloshin S, Schwartz LM, White B, et al. The fate of FDA postapproval studies. *New Engl J Med.* 2017;377(12):1114–1117. doi: 10.1056/NEJMp1705800.

12. FDA Needs to Enhance Its Oversight of Drugs Approved on the Basis of Surrogate Endpoints. In: Testimonies R, ed.: US Government Accountability Office, 2009.

13. Avorn J. The $2.6 billion pill—methodologic and policy considerations. *New Engl J Med.* 2015;372(20):1877–1879. doi: 10.1056/NEJMp1500848.

14. Lu E, Shatzel J, Shin F, et al. What constitutes an "unmet medical need" in oncology? An empirical evaluation of author usage in the biomedical literature. *Semin Oncol.* 2017;44. doi: 10.1053/j.seminoncol.2017.02.009.

15. Yoon SH, Kim KW, Goo JM, et al. Observer variability in RECIST-based tumour burden measurements: a meta-analysis. *Eur J Cancer.* 2016; 53(Supplement C):5–15. doi: https://doi.org/10.1016/j.ejca.2015.10.014.

16. Shao T, Wang L, Templeton AJ, et al. Use and misuse of waterfall plots. *JNl Cancer I.* 2014;106(12). doi: 10.1093/jnci/dju331 [published Online First: 2014 /11/02].

17. Prasad V. Immunotherapy: Tisagenlecleucel—the first approved CAR-T-cell therapy: implications for payers and policy makers. *Nat Rev Clin Oncol.* 2017;advance online publication. doi: 10.1038/nrclinonc.2017.156.

18. Prasad V, Bilal U. The role of censoring on progression free survival: oncologist discretion advised. *Eur J Cancer* 2015;51. doi: 10.1016/j.ejca.2015.07.005.

19. Fojo T, Mailankody S, Lo A. Unintended consequences of expensive cancer therapeutics—the pursuit of marginal indications and a me-too mentality that stifles innovation and creativity: the John Conley lecture. *JAMA Otolaryngol.* 2014;140(12):1225–1236. doi: 10.1001/jamaoto.2014.1570. Accessed August 2, 2019.

20. Prasad V, Vandross A. Failing to improve overall survival because post-protocol survival is long: fact, myth, excuse or improper study design? *J Cancer Res Clin.* 2014;140(4):521–524. doi: 10.1007/s00432–014–1590-x [published Online First: 2014/01/30].

21. Prasad V. The withdrawal of drugs for commercial reasons: the incomplete story of tositumomab. *JAMA Intern Med.* 2014;174(12):1887–1888. doi: 10.1001/jamainternmed.2014.5756.

22. Zia MI, Siu LL, Pond GR, et al. Comparison of outcomes of phase II studies and subsequent randomized control studies using identical chemotherapeutic regimens. *J Clin Oncol.* 2005;23(28):6982–6991. doi: 10.1200/JCo.2005 .06.679.

23. Chen E, Raghunathan V, Prasad V. An overview of cancer drugs approved by the US Food and Drug Administration based on the surrogate end point of response rate. *JAMA Intern Med.* 2019;179(7):915–921. https://jamanetwork .com/journals/jamainternalmedicine/fullarticle/2733563. Accessed August 2, 2019.

Chapter 4. How High Prices Harm Patients and Society

1. Bach PB. Limits on Medicare's ability to control rising spending on cancer drugs. *New Engl J Med.* 2009;360(6):626–633.

2. An unusual business. *Nature Biotechnology.* 2015;33:1113.

3. Prasad V, Wang R, Afifi S, Mailankody S. The rising price of cancer drugs—a new old problem? *JAMA Oncol.* 2017;3(2):277–278.

4. DiMasi JA, Grabowski HG. Economics of new oncology drug development. *J Clin Oncol.* 2007;25(2):209–216.

5. Mattina J, Carlisle B, Hachem Y, Fergusson D, Kimmelman J. Inefficiencies and patient burdens in the development of the targeted cancer drug sorafenib: a systematic review. *PLoS Biology.* 2017;15(2):e2000487.

6. Neumann PJ, Cohen JT, Weinstein MC. Updating cost-effectiveness—the curious resilience of the $50,000-per-QALY threshold. *New Engl J Med.* 2014; 371(9):796–797.

7. Saret CJ, Winn AN, Shah G, et al. Value of innovation in hematologic malignancies: a systematic review of published cost-effectiveness analyses. *Blood.* 2015;125(12):1866–1869.

8. Prasad V, Mailankody S. How should we assess the value of innovative drugs in oncology? lessons from cost-effectiveness analyses. *Blood.* 2015;126(15):1860–1861.

9. Bell CM, Urbach DR, Ray JG, et al. Bias in published cost effectiveness studies: systematic review. *BMJ.* 2006;332(7543):699–703.

10. Prasad V. The apples and oranges of cost-effectiveness. *Clev Clin J Med.* 2012;79(6):377–379.

11. Howard, D, Bach P, Berndt E, Conti R. 2015. Pricing in the market for anticancer drugs. *JEP.* 29(1):139–162.

12. Bach PB. New Math on Drug Cost-Effectiveness. *New Engl J Med.* 2015; 373(19):1797–1799.

13. Prasad V. Immunotherapy: Tisagenlecleucel—the first approved CAR-T-cell therapy: implications for payers and policy makers. *Nat Rev Clin Oncol.* 2017; advance online publication.

14. Neelapu SS, Tummala S, Kebriaei P, et al. Chimeric antigen receptor T-cell therapy—assessment and management of toxicities. *Nat Rev Clin Oncol.* 2018; 15(1):47–62.

15. @PlenarySessShow. Oh finally, FDA gives the intention to treat response rate of CAR T Tisa. Right column. #ASH17. 2017; https://twitter.com/PlenarySess Show/status/939973679617925120. Accessed September 5, 2018.

16. Altman J, Hasserjian RP, Burns LJ, Wiley K. AML MATTERS: a multidisciplinary approach to testing and diagnosis, evaluation of risk, and personalized treatment selection. Paper presented at the American Society of Hematology (ASH) Annual Meeting, 2017.

17. Novartis pivotal CTL019 6-month follow-up data show durable remission rates in children, young adults with r/r B-cell ALL [press release]. [Online], June 23, 2017.

18. Prasad V. Immunotherapy: tisagenlecleucel—the first approved CAR-T-cell therapy: implications for payers and policy makers. *Nat Rev Clin Oncol.* 2018; 15(1):11–12.

19. Grady D. In girl's last hope, altered immune cells beat leukemia. *New York Times.* December. 9, 2012;Health

20. Hernandez I, Prasad V, Gellad WF. Total costs of chimeric antigen receptor t-cell immunotherapy. *JAMA Oncol.* 2018;1;4(7):994–996.

Chapter 5. Hype, Spin, and the Unbridled Enthusiasm That Distorts Cancer Medicine

1. Bowles HJ, Clarke KL. Palbociclib: a new option for front-line treatment of metastatic, hormone receptor–positive, HER2-negative breast cancer. *J AdvPract Oncol.* 2015;6(6):577–581.

2. Spencer B. Hope for breast cancer patients as "game changing" new treatment could delay gruelling chemotherapy for months. 2016; http://www.dailymail .co.uk/health/article-3473423/Hope-breast-cancer-patients-game-changing-new -treatment-delay-gruelling-chemotherapy-months.html. Accessed October 25, 2017.

3. Graham CM, 2016. "Game-changing" breast cancer treatment delays growth of tumour. *Health News,* 2016; http://www.telegraph.co.uk/news/health/news /12181741/Game-changing-breast-cancer-treatment-delays-growth-of-tumour .html. Accessed October 25, 2017.

4. Feek B. "Cancer drug available to New Zealand women who can afford it." *Breast Cancer* [Internet]. 2017; http://www.scmp.com/news/asia/australasia /article/2109670/breast-cancer-game-changer-hits-new-zealand-only-women-who -can. Accessed October 25, 2017.

5. Abola MV, Prasad V. The use of superlatives in cancer research. *JAMA Oncol.* 2016;2(1):139–141.

6. Blagoev KB, Wilkerson J, Fojo T. Hazard ratios in cancer clinical trials—a primer. *Nat Rev Clin Oncol.* 2012;9(3):178–183.

7. Tayapongsak Duggan K, De Jesus K, Kemp R, Prasad V. Use of word "unprecedented" in the media coverage of cancer drugs: Do "unprecedented" drugs live up to the hype? *J Cancer Policy.* 2017;14:16–20.

8. Easson EC, Russell MH. Cure of Hodgkin's Disease. *Br Med J.* 1963;1(5347): 1704–1707.

9. Pope A. *An Essay on Man: In Four Epistles, to Henry St. John, L. Boling-*

broke. Philadelphia: Printed for Thomas Dobson, at the stone house, no. 41, South, Second-Street.1792.

10. FDA Commissioner Scott Gottlieb calls approval of the first U.S. cancer gene therapy "a significant milestone." *Washington Post*; 2017. https://www .washingtonpost.com/blogs/post-live/wp/2017/09/19/fda-commissioner-scott -gottlieb-calls-approval-of-the-first-u-s-cancer-gene-therapy-a-significant-mile stone/?utm_term=.12c2012defea. Accessed October 25.

11. Kolata G. Leading cancer experts comment on the cancer initiative in the state of the union address. *AACR Press Office* 2016; http://blog.aacr.org/leading -cancer-experts-comment-on-the-cancer-initiative-in-the-state-of-the-union -address/. Accessed October 25, 2017.

12. Kopans DB. More misinformation on breast cancer screening. *Gland Surgery.* 2017;6(1):125–129.

13. Von Eschenbach AC. NCI sets goal of eliminating suffering and death due to cancer by 2015. *J Natl Med Assoc.* 2003;95(7):637–639.

14. Rosenthal ET. Andrew von Eschenbach and the cancer cure—former NCI and FDA head admits he made a mistake. *Health Policy* 2016; https://www.med pagetoday.com/publichealthpolicy/healthpolicy/58881. Accessed October 25, 2017.

15. Vera-Badillo FE, Shapiro R, Ocana A, Amir E, Tannock IF. Bias in report-ing of end points of efficacy and toxicity in randomized, clinical trials for women with breast cancer. *Ann Oncol.* 2013;24(5):1238–1244.

16. Boutron I, Altman DG, Hopewell S, Vera-Badillo F, Tannock I, Ravaud P. Impact of spin in the abstracts of articles reporting results of randomized con-trolled trials in the field of cancer: the SPIIN randomized controlled trial. *J Clin Oncol.* 2014;32(36):4120–4126.

17. Positive results from phase III ECHELON-1 trial evaluating brentuximab vedotin in frontline advanced hodgkin lymphoma. InPress Media Group, LLC, 2017. https://adcreview.com/news/positive-results-phase-iii-echelon-1-trial-eval uating-brentuximab-vedotin-frontline-advanced-hodgkin-lymphoma/. Accessed October 25, 2017.

18. @DrMatasar. "Ask us once we've seen data, not press releases." 2017; https://twitter.com/DrMatasar/status/917508362773893121.

19. Celgene will discontinue phase III ORIGIN® trial in previously untreated elderly patients with B-cell chronic lymphocytic leukemia [press release]. Summit, NJ: Business Wire, July 18, 2013.

20. Chanan-Khan A, Egyed M, Robak T, et al. Randomized phase 3 study of lenalidomide versus chlorambucil as first-line therapy for older patients with chronic lymphocytic leukemia (the ORIGIN trial). *Leukemia.* 2017;31(5):1240–1243.

21. Ioannidis JA. Are medical conferences useful? And for whom? *JAMA.* 2012;307(12):1257–1258.

22. Massey PR, Wang R, Prasad V, Bates SE, Fojo T. Assessing the eventual publication of clinical trial abstracts submitted to a large annual oncology meeting. *Oncologist.* 2016;21(3):261–268.

23. Booth CM, Le Maitre A, Ding K, et al. Presentation of nonfinal results of randomized controlled trials at major oncology meetings *J Clin Oncol.* 2009;27(24):3938–3944.

Chapter 6. Financial Conflict of Interest

1. Marshall DC, Moy B, Jackson ME, Mackey TK, Hattangadi-Gluth JA. Distribution and patterns of industry-related payments to oncologists in 2014. *JNCI: J Natl Cancer I.* 2016;108(12):djw163-djw163.

2. Green AK, Wood WA, Basch EM. Time to reassess the cancer compendia for off-label drug coverage in oncology. *JAMA.* 2016;316(15):1541–1542.

3. Mitchell AP, Basch EM, Dusetzina SB. Financial relationships with industry among national comprehensive cancer network guideline authors. *JAMA Oncol.* 2016;2(12):1628–1631.

4. Boothby A, Wang R, Cetnar J, Prasad V. Effect of the American society of clinical oncology's conflict of interest policy on information overload. *JAMA Oncol.* 2016;2(12):1653–1654.

5. @VPrasadMDMPH. @JatinShahMD think you are still sore about my slide (below). don't worry lots of docs owe career to pharma [tweet]. 2016; https://twitter.com/VPrasadMDMPH/status/730907035449982977.

6. Tao DL, Boothby A, McLouth J, Prasad V. Financial conflicts of interest among hematologist-oncologists on Twitter. *JAMA Intern Med.* 2017;177(3): 425–427.

7. Kaestner V, Brown A, Tao D, Prasad V. Conflicts of interest in Twitter. *Lancet Haematology.* 2017;4(9):e408–e409.

8. Patient groups funded by drugmakers are largely mum on high drug prices. *USA Today* 2016. https://www.usatoday.com/story/news/nation/2016/01/21/patient-groups-drug-makers-high-drug-prices/79001722/. Accessed November 1, 2017.

9. Patients for Affordable Drugs. https://www.patientsforaffordabledrugs.org/.

10. Abola MV, Prasad V. Industry funding of cancer patient advocacy organizations. *Mayo Clin Proc.* 91(11):1668–1670.

11. Bien J, Prasad V. Future jobs of FDA's haematology-oncology reviewers. *BMJ.* 2016;354.

12. Prasad V. Who is right: Bien and I or employees of the US FDA? *BMJ.* 2016;354:i5055.

13. Piller C. Is FDA's revolving door open too wide? *Science.* 2018;361(6397):21.

14. Lurie P, Almeida CM, Stine N, Stine AR, Wolfe SM. Financial conflict of interest disclosure and voting patterns at Food and Drug Administration drug advisory committee meetings. *JAMA.* 2006;295(16):1921–1928.

15. Tibau A, Ocana A, Anguera G, et al. Oncologic drugs advisory committee recommendations and approval of cancer drugs by the US Food and Drug Administration. *JAMA Oncol.* 2016;2(6):744–750.

16. Xu J, Emenanjo O, Ortwerth M, Lurie P. Association of appearance of conflicts of interest with voting behavior at FDA Advisory Committee meetings—a cross-sectional study. *JAMA Intern Med.* 2017;177(7):1038–1040.

17. Lammers A, Edmiston J, Kaestner V, Prasad V. Financial conflict of interest and academic influence among experts speaking on behalf of the pharmaceutical industry at the US Food and Drug Administration's oncologic drugs advisory committee meetings. *Mayo Clin Proc.* 2017;92(7):1164–1166.

18. Graham SS, Card DJ, Ahn S, Kim SY, Kessler MM, Olson MK. Conflicts of

interest among patient and consumer representatives to U.S. Food and Drug Administration drug advisory committees. *Ann Intern Med.* 2016;165(8):606–607.

19. Abola MV, Prasad V. Characteristics and conflicts of public speakers at meetings of the oncologic drugs advisory committee to the US Food and Drug Administration. *JAMA Intern Med.* 2016;176(3):389–391.

Chapter 7. The Harms of Financial Conflicts and How to Rehabilitate Medicine

1. De Jesus-Morales K, Prasad V. Closed financial loops: when they happen in government, they're called corruption; in medicine, they're just a footnote. *Hastings Center Report.* 2017;47(3):9–14.

2. Powell L. Ex-Va. governor Robert McDonnell guilty of 11 counts of corruption. *Washinigton Post.* September 4, 2014;Virgina Politics.

3. Toobin J. The showman: how U.S. attorney Preet Bharara struck fear into Wall Street and Albany. In: *The New Yorker.* May 2, 2016. https://www.new yorker.com/magazine/2016/05/09/the-man-who-terrifies-wall-street. Accessed August 2, 2019.

4. Fleischman W, Agrawal S, King M, et al. Association between payments from manufacturers of pharmaceuticals to physicians and regional prescribing: cross sectional ecological study. *BMJ.* 2016;354.

5. Yeh JS, Franklin JM, Avorn J, Landon J, Kesselheim AS. Association of industry payments to physicians with the prescribing of brand-name statins in massachusetts. *JAMA Int Med.* 2016;176(6):763–768.

6. DeJong C, Aguilar T, Tseng C, Lin GA, Boscardin W, Dudley R. Pharmaceutical industry–sponsored meals and physician prescribing patterns for medicare beneficiaries. *JAMA Intern Med.* 2016;176(8):1114–1122.

7. Wang AT, McCoy CP, Murad MH, Montori VM. Association between industry affiliation and position on cardiovascular risk with rosiglitazone: cross sectional systematic review. *BMJ.* 2010;340.

8. Fugh-Berman A, McDonald CP, Bell AM, Bethards EC, Scialli AR. Promotional tone in reviews of menopausal hormone therapy after the Women's Health Initiative: an analysis of published articles. *PLoS Medicine.* 2011;8(3):e1000425.

9. Ornstein CaT, K. Top Cancer researcher fails to disclose corporate financial ties in major research journals. *New York Times.* September 8, 2018;Health.

10. Thomas KaO, C. Top Sloan Kettering cancer doctor resigns after failing to disclose industry ties. *New York Times.* September 13, 2018;Health.

11. Boothby A, Wang R, Cetnar J, Prasad V. Effect of the American Society of Clinical Oncology's conflict of interest policy on information overload: ASCO's conflict of interest policy and information overload letters. *JAMA Oncol.* 2016; 2(12):1653–1654.

12. Kaestner V, Edmiston JB, Prasad V. The relation between publication rate and financial conflict of interest among physician authors of high-impact oncology publications: an observational study. *CMAJ Open.* 2018;6(1):e57–e62.

13. Ornstein C. New England Journal of Medicine increasingly targeted by critics. *Boston Globe.* April 5, 2016.

14. Relman AS. The new medical-industrial complex. *New Engl J Med.* 1980; 303(17):963–970.

15. Kassirer J. *Unanticipated Outcomes: A Medical Memoir.* Independent (self published); 2017.

16. Steinbrook R, Kassirer JP, Angell M. Justifying conflicts of interest in medical journals: a very bad idea. *BMJ.* 2015;350:h2942.

17. Kaestner V, Prasad V. Financial conflicts of interest among editorialists in high-impact journals. *Blood Cancer J.* 2017;7:e611.

18. Prasad V, Rajkumar SV. Conflict of interest in academic oncology: moving beyond the blame game and forging a path forward. *Blood Cancer J.* 2016;6:e489.

Chapter 8. Will Precision Oncology Save Us?

1. Jha A. In conversation with . . . Harold Varmus. Alok Jha talks to Harold Varmus, Nobel Prize–winning cancer researcher and current director of the US National Cancer Institute. *Story.* 2014; https://mosaicscience.com/story/conversation-with-harold-varmus. Accessed November 15, 2017.

2. Prasad V., Gale RG. What precisely is precision oncology—and will it work? 2017; http://www.ascopost.com/issues/january-25–2017/what-precisely-is-precision-oncology-and-will-it-work/. Accessed November 15, 2017.

3. Lu E, Shatzel J, Shin F, Prasad V. What constitutes an "unmet medical need" in oncology? An empirical evaluation of author usage in the biomedical literature. *Semin Oncol.* 2017;44.

4. Foundation Medicine announces 2016 second quarter results and recent highlights [press release]. August 2, 2016.

5. Teichert E. Innovations: startup's liquid biopsies match cancer patients with trials. *Medical Equipment.* 2016; http://www.modernhealthcare.com/article/20160820/MAGAZINE/308209978. Accessed November 15, 2017.

6. Fernandes D. United Health agrees to cover genetic cancer test from Foundation Medicine. *Boston Globe.* December 21, 2015;Business.

7. National Cancer Insititute. Update: NCI Formulary & NCI-MATCH Trial. https://deainfo.nci.nih.gov/advisory/bsa/0317/Doroshow.pdf. Published March 21, 2017. Accessed August 2, 2019.

8. Wheler JJ, Janku F, Naing A, et al. Cancer therapy directed by comprehensive genomic profiling: a single center study. *Cancer Res.* 2016;76(13):3690–3701.

9. Kuderer NM, Burton KA, Blau S, et al. Comparison of 2 commercially available next-generation sequencing platforms in oncology. *JAMA Oncol.* 2017; 3(7):996–998.

10. Hahn AW, Gill DM, Maughan B, et al. Correlation of genomic alterations assessed by next-generation sequencing (NGS) of tumor tissue DNA and circulating tumor DNA (ctDNA) in metastatic renal cell carcinoma (mRCC): potential clinical implications. *Oncotarget.* 2017;8(20):33614–33620.

11. Chae YK, Davis AA, Carneiro BA, et al. Concordance between genomic alterations assessed by next-generation sequencing in tumor tissue or circulating cell-free DNA. *Oncotarget.* 2016;7(40):65364–65373.

12. Weiss GJ, Hoff BR, Whitehead RP, et al. Evaluation and comparison of two commercially available targeted next-generation sequencing platforms to assist oncology decision making. *OncoTargets Ther.* 2015;8:959–967.

13. Prasad V, Vandross A. Characteristics of exceptional or super responders to cancer drugs. *Mayo Clin Proc.* 2015;90(12):1639–1649.

14. Nishikawa G, Luo J, Prasad V. A comprehensive review of exceptional responders to anticancer drugs in the biomedical literature. *Eur J Cancer.* 2018; 101:143–151.

15. Le Tourneau C, Delord JP, Goncalves A, et al. Molecularly targeted therapy based on tumour molecular profiling versus conventional therapy for advanced cancer (SHIVA): a multicentre, open-label, proof-of-concept, randomised, controlled phase 2 trial. *Lancet Oncol.* 2015;16(13):1324–1334.

16. Schwaederle M, Zhao M, Lee JJ, et al. Impact of precision medicine in diverse cancers: a meta-analysis of phase II clinical trials. *J Clin Oncol.* 2015; 33(32):3817–3825.

17. Schwaederle M, Zhao M, Lee JJ, et al. Association of biomarker-based treatment strategies with response rates and progression-free survival in refractory malignant neoplasms: a meta-analysis. *JAMA Oncol.* 2016;2(11):1452–1459.

Chapter 9. Study Design 201

1. Thompson D. Are nuts good medicine for colon cancer survivors? *Colorectal Cancer* 2017; https://www.webmd.com/colorectal-cancer/news/20170517/nuts -good-medicine-for-colon-cancer-survivors#1. Accessed September 18, 2018.

2. Steenhuysen J. Eating tree nuts may cut risk that colon cancer will return: study. 2017; https://www.reuters.com/article/us-health-cancer-nuts/eating-tree -nuts-may-cut-risk-that-colon-cancer-will-return-study-idUSKCN18D2P8. Accessed September 18, 2018.

3. Efficacy of adjuvant fluorouracil and folinic acid in colon cancer: interna- tional multicentre pooled analysis of colon cancer trials (IMPACT) investigators. *Lancet.* 1995;345(8955):939–944.

4. Andre T, Boni C, Navarro M, et al. Improved overall survival with oxalipla- tin, fluorouracil, and leucovorin as adjuvant treatment in stage II or III colon cancer in the MOSAIC trial. *J Clin Oncol.* 2009;27(19):3109–3116.

5. Allegra CJ, Yothers G, O'Connell MJ, et al. Bevacizumab in stage II–III colon cancer: 5-year update of the National Surgical Adjuvant Breast and Bowel Project C-08 trial. *J Clin Oncol.* 2013;31(3):359–364.

6. Allegra CJ, Yothers G, O'Connell MJ, et al. Initial safety report of NSABP C-08: a randomized phase III study of modified FOLFOX6 with or without bevacizumab for the adjuvant treatment of patients with stage II or III colon cancer. *J Clin Oncol.* 2009;27(20):3385–3390.

7. de Gramont A, Van Cutsem E, Schmoll HJ, et al. Bevacizumab plus oxaliplatin-based chemotherapy as adjuvant treatment for colon cancer (AVANT): a phase 3 randomised controlled trial. *Lancet Oncol.* 2012;13(12):1225–1233.

8. Kerr RS, Love S, Segelov E, et al. Adjuvant capecitabine plus bevacizumab versus capecitabine alone in patients with colorectal cancer (QUASAR 2): an open- label, randomised phase 3 trial. *Lancet Oncol.* 2016;17(11):1543–1557.

9. Saltz LB, Niedzwiecki D, Hollis D, et al. Irinotecan fluorouracil plus leuco- vorin is not superior to fluorouracil plus leucovorin alone as adjuvant treatment for stage III colon cancer: results of CALGB 89803. *J Clin Oncol.* 2007;25(23):3456– 3461.

10. Van Cutsem E, Labianca R, Bodoky G, et al. Randomized phase III trial comparing biweekly infusional fluorouracil/leucovorin alone or with irinotecan in

the adjuvant treatment of stage III colon cancer: PETACC-3. *J Clin Oncol.* 2009; 27(19):3117–3125.

11. Ychou M, Raoul JL, Douillard JY, et al. A phase III randomised trial of LV5FU2 + irinotecan versus LV5FU2 alone in adjuvant high-risk colon cancer (FNCLCC Accord02/FFCD9802). *Ann Oncol.* 2009;20(4):674–680.

12. Alberts SR, Sargent DJ, Nair S, et al. Effect of oxaliplatin, fluorouracil, and leucovorin with or without cetuximab on survival among patients with resected stage III colon cancer: a randomized trial. *JAMA.* 2012;307(13):1383–1393.

13. Taieb J, Balogoun R, Le Malicot K, et al. Adjuvant FOLFOX +/– cetuximab in full RAS and BRAF wildtype stage III colon cancer patients. *Ann Oncol.* 2017; 28(4):824–830.

14. Fadelu T, Zhang S, Niedzwiecki D, et al. Nut consumption and survival in patients with stage III colon cancer: results rom CALGB 89803 (Alliance). *J Clin Oncol.* 2018;36(11):1112–1120.

15. Derrick L, Tao NDG, Prasad V. Statistical significance of bevacizumab trials when considering the portfolio of all studies. *2018 ASCO Annual Meeting J Clin Oncol 36, 2018 (suppl; abstr 6551).* 2018.

16. Patel CJ, Burford B, Ioannidis JP. Assessment of vibration of effects due to model specification can demonstrate the instability of observational associations. *J Clin Epidemiol.* 2015;68(9):1046–1058.

17. Grothey A, Sugrue MM, Purdie DM, et al. Bevacizumab beyond first progression is associated with prolonged overall survival in metastatic colorectal cancer: results from a large observational cohort study (BRiTE). *J Clin Oncol.* 2008;26(33):5326–5334.

18. Hirschtick R. Extremities. *JAMA.* 2008;300(10):1125–1126.

19. Stanbrook MB, Austin PC, Redelmeier DA. Acronym-named randomized trials in medicine—the ART in medicine study. *New Engl J Med.* 2006;355(1): 101–102.

20. Bennouna J, Sastre J, Arnold D, et al. Continuation of bevacizumab after first progression in metastatic colorectal cancer (ML18147): a randomised phase 3 trial. *Lancet Oncol.* 14(1):29–37.

21. Fisher RI, Gaynor ER, Dahlberg S, et al. Comparison of a standard regimen (CHOP) with three intensive chemotherapy regimens for advanced non-Hodgkin's lymphoma. *New Engl J Med.* 1993;328(14):1002–1006.

22. Fisher RI, Longo DL, DeVita VT, Jr., Hubbard SM, Miller TP, Young RC. Long-term follow-up of ProMACE-CytaBOM in non-Hodgkin's lymphomas. *Ann Oncol.* 1991;2 Suppl 1:33–35.

23. Miller TP, Dahlberg S, Weick JK, et al. Unfavorable histologies of non-Hodgkin's lymphoma treated with ProMACE-CytaBOM: a groupwide Southwest Oncology Group study. *J Clin Oncol.* 1990;8(12):1951–1958.

24. Sacks H, Chalmers TC, Smith H, Jr. Randomized versus historical controls for clinical trials. *Am J Med.* 1982;72(2):233–240.

25. Zia MI, Siu LL, Pond GR, Chen EX. Comparison of outcomes of phase II studies and subsequent randomized control studies using identical chemotherapeutic regimens. *J Clin Oncol.* 2005;23(28):6982–6991.

26. Prasad V. Double-crossed: why crossover in clinical trials may be distorting medical science. *J Natl Compr Canc Net: JNCCN.* 2013;11(5):625–627.

27. Prasad V, Grady C. The misguided ethics of crossover trials. *Contemp Clin Trials.* 2014;37(2):167–169.

28. Haslam A, Prasad V. When is crossover desirable in cancer drug trials and when is it problematic? *Ann Oncol.* 2018;29(5):1079–1081.

29. Reck M, Rodríguez-Abreu D, Robinson AG, et al. Pembrolizumab versus chemotherapy for PD-L1–positive non-small-cell lung cancer. *New Engl J Med.* 2016;375(19):1823–1833.

30. Fizazi K, Tran N, Fein L, et al. Abiraterone plus prednisone in metastatic, castration-sensitive prostate cancer. *New Engl J Med.* 2017;377(4):352–360.

31. Chen EY, Prasad V. Crossover is not associated with faster trial accrual. *Ann Oncol.* 2018;29(3):776–777.

32. Kantoff PW, Higano CS, Shore ND, et al. Sipuleucel-T immunotherapy for castration-resistant prostate cancer. *New Engl J Med.* 2010;363(5):411–422.

33. Mark D, Samson DJ, Bonnell CJ, Ziegler KM, Aronson N. AHRQ Technology Assessments. In: *Outcomes of Sipuleucel-T Therapy.* Rockville, MD: Agency for Healthcare Research and Quality (US); 2011.

34. Mulcahy N. Futile: prostate cancer vaccine phase 3 trial ends. *Oncology News* 2017; https://www.medscape.com/viewarticle/885877. Accessed September 18, 2018.

35. Schlumberger M, Elisei R, Müller S, et al. Overall survival analysis of EXAM, a phase III trial of cabozantinib in patients with radiographically progressive medullary thyroid carcinoma. *Ann Oncol.* 2017;28(11):2813–2819.

36. Leboulleux S, Bastholt L, Krause T, et al. Vandetanib in locally advanced or metastatic differentiated thyroid cancer: a randomised, double-blind, phase 2 trial. *Lancet Oncol.* 2012;13(9):897–905.

37. CAPRELSA® (vandetanib) [package insert]. AstraZeneca Pharmaceuticals LP: Wilmington, DE; 2011.

38. Moore TJ, Furberg CD. The safety risks of innovation: the FDA's expedited drug development pathway. *JAMA.* 2012;308(9):869–870.

39. Kay A, Higgins J, Day AG, Meyer RM, Booth CM. Randomized controlled trials in the era of molecular oncology: methodology, biomarkers, and end points. *Ann Oncol.* 2012;23.

40. Moore MJ, Goldstein D, Hamm J, et al. Erlotinib plus gemcitabine compared with gemcitabine alone in patients with advanced pancreatic cancer: a phase III trial of the National Cancer Institute of Canada Clinical Trials Group. *J Clin Oncol.* 2007;25(15):1960–1966.

41. Kimmelman J, Carlisle B, Gönen M. Drug development at the portfolio level is important for policy, care decisions and human protections. *JAMA.* 2017; 318(11):1003–1004.

42. Brawley L. With 20 agents, 803 trials, and 166,736 patient slots, is pharma investing too heavily in PD-1 drug development? *Cancer Letter.* 2016;42(37).

Chapter 10. Principles of Oncology Practice

1. Saltz LB, Niedzwiecki D, Hollis D, et al. Irinotecan fluorouracil plus leucovorin is not superior to fluorouracil plus leucovorin alone as adjuvant treatment for stage III colon cancer: results of CALGB 89803. *J Clin Oncol.* 2007;25(23): 3456–3461.

2. Bruix J, Takayama T, Mazzaferro V, et al. Adjuvant sorafenib for hepato-cellular carcinoma after resection or ablation (STORM): a phase 3, randomised, double-blind, placebo-controlled trial. *Lancet Oncol.*16(13):1344–1354.

3. de Gramont A, Van Cutsem E, Schmoll H-J, et al. Bevacizumab plus oxaliplatin-based chemotherapy as adjuvant treatment for colon cancer (AVANT): a phase 3 randomised controlled trial. *Lancet Oncol.*13(12):1225–1233.

4. Pogue-Geile K, Yothers G, Taniyama Y, et al. Defective mismatch repair and benefit from bevacizumab for colon cancer: findings from NSABP C-08. *JNCI: J Natl Cancer I.* 2013;105(13):989–992.

5. Group QC. Adjuvant chemotherapy versus observation in patients with colorectal cancer: a randomised study. *Lancet.* 370(9604):2020–2029.

6. Kerr RS, Love S, Segelov E, et al. Adjuvant capecitabine plus bevacizumab versus capecitabine alone in patients with colorectal cancer (QUASAR 2): an open-label, randomised phase 3 trial. *Lancet Oncol.* 17(11):1543–1557.

7. Alberts SR, Sinicrope FA, Grothey A. No147: A randomized phase III trial of oxaliplatin plus 5-Fluorouracil/leucovorin with or without cetuximab after curative resection of stage III colon cancer. *Clin Colorectal Canc.* 2005;5(3): 211–213.

8. Taieb J, Tabernero J, Mini E, et al. Oxaliplatin, fluorouracil, and leucovorin with or without cetuximab in patients with resected stage III colon cancer (PETACC-8): an open-label, randomised phase 3 trial. *Lancet Oncol.*15(8): 862–873.

9. Kelly K, Altorki NK, Eberhardt WEE, et al. Adjuvant erlotinib versus placebo in patients with stage IB-IIIA non-small-cell lung cancer (RADIANT): a randomized, double-blind, hase III trial. *J Clin Oncol.* 2015;33(34):4007–4014.

10. Goss PE, Smith IE, O'Shaughnessy J, et al. Adjuvant lapatinib for women with early-stage HER2-positive breast cancer: a randomised, controlled, phase 3 trial. *Lancet Oncol.* 2013;14(1):88–96.

11. McCullough AE, Dell'Orto P, Reinholz MM, et al. Central pathology laboratory review of HER2 and ER in early breast cancer: an ALTTO trial [BIG 2-06/NCCTG No63D (Alliance)] ring study. *Breast Cancer Res Tr.* 2014;143(3): 485–492.

12. Gyawali B, Ando Y. Adjuvant sunitinib for high-risk-resected renal cell carcinoma: a meta-analysis of ASSURE and S-TRAC trials. *Ann Oncol.* 2017; 28(4):898–899.

13. Haas NB, Manola J, Uzzo RG, et al. Adjuvant sunitinib or sorafenib for high-risk, non-metastatic renal-cell carcinoma (ECOG-ACRIN E2805): a double-blind, placebo-controlled, randomised, phase 3 trial. *Lancet.* 2016;387(10032): 2008–2016.

14. Ravaud A, Motzer RJ, Pandha HS, et al. Adjuvant sunitinib in high-risk renal-cell carcinoma after nephrectomy. *New Engl J Med.* 2016;375(23):2246–2254.

15. Prasad V, Kim C, Burotto M, Vandross A. The strength of association between surrogate end points and survival in oncology: a systematic review of trial-level meta-analyses. *JAMA Intern Med.* 2015;175(8):1389–1398.

16. Ebata T, Hirano S, Konishi M, et al. Randomized clinical trial of adjuvant

gemcitabine chemotherapy versus observation in resected bile duct cancer. *Br J Surg.* 2018;105(3):192–202.

17. Eisenhauer EA, Therasse P, Bogaerts J, et al. New response evaluation criteria in solid tumours: revised RECIST guideline (version 1.1). *Eur J Cancer.* 2009;45(2):228–247.

18. Burotto M, Wilkerson J, Stein W, Motzer R, Bates S, Fojo T. Continuing a cancer treatment despite tumor growth may be valuable: sunitinib in renal cell carcinoma as example. *PLOS ONE.* 2014;9(5):e96316.

19. Larkin J, Chiarion-Sileni V, Gonzalez R, et al. Combined nivolumab and ipilimumab or monotherapy in untreated melanoma. *New Engl J Med.* 2015; 373(1):23–34.

20. Hanna NH, Sandier AB, Loehrer PJ, Sr., et al. Maintenance daily oral etoposide versus no further therapy following induction chemotherapy with etoposide plus ifosfamide plus cisplatin in extensive small-cell lung cancer: a Hoosier Oncology Group randomized study. *Ann Oncol.* 2002;13(1):95–102.

21. Sledge GW, Neuberg D, Bernardo P, et al. Phase III Trial of doxorubicin, paclitaxel, and the combination of doxorubicin and paclitaxel as front-line chemotherapy for metastatic breast cancer: an intergroup trial (E1193). *J Clin Oncol.* 2003;21(4):588–592.

22. Rini BI, Dorff TB, Elson P, et al. Active surveillance in metastatic renal-cell carcinoma: a prospective, phase 2 trial. *Lancet Oncol.* 2016;17(9):1317–1324.

23. Brice P, Bastion Y, Lepage E, et al. Comparison in low-tumor-burden follicular lymphomas between an initial no-treatment policy, prednimustine, or interferon alfa: a randomized study from the Groupe d'Etude des Lymphomes Folliculaires. Groupe d'Etude des Lymphomes de l'Adulte. *J Clin Oncol.* 1997; 15(3):1110–1117.

24. Ardeshna KM, Smith P, Norton A, et al. Long-term effect of a watch and wait policy versus immediate systemic treatment for asymptomatic advanced-stage non-Hodgkin lymphoma: a randomised controlled trial. *Lancet.* 2003;362(9383): 516–522.

25. Horning SJ, Rosenberg SA. The natural history of initially untreated low-grade non-Hodgkin's lymphomas. *New Engl J Med.* 1984;311(23):1471–1475.

26. O'Brien ME, Easterbrook P, Powell J, et al. The natural history of low grade non-Hodgkin's lymphoma and the impact of a no initial treatment policy on survival. *Q J Med.* 1991;80(292):651–660.

27. Gattiker HH, Wiltshaw E, Galton DA. Spontaneous regression in non-Hodgkin's lymphoma. *Cancer.* 1980;45(10):2627–2632.

28. Krikorian JG, Portlock CS, Cooney P, Rosenberg SA. Spontaneous regression of non-Hodgkin's lymphoma: a report of nine cases. *Cancer.* 1980;46(9): 2093–2099.

29. Solal-Celigny P, Bellei M, Marcheselli L, et al. Watchful waiting in low-tumor burden follicular lymphoma in the rituximab era: results of an F2-study database. *J Clin Oncol.* 2012;30(31):3848–3853.

30. Ackland SP, Jones M, Tu D, et al. A meta-analysis of two randomised trials of early chemotherapy in asymptomatic metastatic colorectal cancer. *Brit J Cancer.* 2005;93:1236.

31. Prasad V. But how many people died? health outcomes in perspective. *Clev Clin J Med.* 2015;82(3):146–150.

Chapter 11. Important Trials in Oncology

1. Vandross A, Prasad V, Mailankody S. ASCO plenary sessions: impact, legacy, future. *Semin Oncol.* 2016;43(3):321–326.

2. Rustin GJ, van der Burg ME, Griffin CL, et al. Early versus delayed treatment of relapsed ovarian cancer (MRC OV05/EORTC 55955): a randomised trial. *Lancet.* 2010;376(9747):1155–1163.

3. Rustin GJS, van der Burg MEL, Griffin CL, et al. Early versus delayed treatment of relapsed ovarian cancer (MRC OV05/EORTC 55955): a randomised trial. *Lancet.* 2010;376(9747):1155–1163.

4. Esselen KM, Cronin AM, Bixel K, et al. Use of ca-125 tests and computed tomographic scans for surveillance in ovarian cancer. *JAMA Oncol.* 2016;2(11): 1427–1433.

5. Soulos PR, Yu JB, Roberts KB, et al. Assessing the impact of a cooperative group trial on breast cancer care in the medicare population. *J Clin Oncol.* 2012; 30(14):1601–1607.

6. McCormick B, Ottesen RA, Hughes ME, et al. Impact of guideline changes on use or omission of radiation in the elderly with early breast cancer: practice patterns at national comprehensive cancer network institutions. *J Am Coll Surgeons.* 2014;219(4):796–802.

7. Mulcahy N. The "fatal attraction" of an ovarian cancer test. *News Oncology* 2016; https://www.medscape.com/viewarticle/867650. Accessed January 11, 2018.

8. Buys SS, Partridge E, Black A, et al. Effect of screening on ovarian cancer mortality: the prostate, lung, colorectal and ovarian (PLCO) cancer screening randomized controlled trial. *JAMA.* 2011;305(22):2295–2303.

9. Jacobs IJ, Parmar M, Skates SJ, Menon U. Ovarian cancer screening: UKCTOCS trial—authors' reply. *Lancet.* 2016;387(10038):2603–2604.

10. Metro G, Chiari R, Baldi A, De Angelis V, Minotti V, Crinò L. Selumetinib: a promising pharmacologic approach for KRAS-mutant advanced non-small-cell lung cancer. *Future Oncology.* 2013;9(2):167–177.

11. Jänne PA, van den Heuvel MM, Barlesi F, et al. Selumetinib plus docetaxel compared with docetaxel alone and progression-free survival in patients with kras-mutant advanced non-small cell lung cancer: the select-1 randomized clinical trial. *JAMA.* 2017;317(18):1844–1853.

12. O'Shaughnessy J, Osborne C, Pippen JE, et al. Iniparib plus chemotherapy in metastatic triple-negative breast cancer. *New Engl J Med.* 2011;364(3):205–214.

13. O'Shaughnessy J, Schwartzberg L, Danso MA, et al. Phase III study of iniparib plus gemcitabine and carboplatin versus gemcitabine and carboplatin in patients with metastatic triple-negative breast cancer. *J Clin Oncol.* 2014;32(34): 3840–3847.

14. Kantoff PW, Schuetz TJ, Blumenstein BA, et al. Overall survival analysis of a phase II randomized controlled trial of a poxviral-based PSA-targeted immunotherapy in metastatic castration-resistant prostate cancer. *J Clin Oncol.* 2010; 28(7):1099–1105.

15. Prostvac. 2017; https://en.wikipedia.org/wiki/Prostvac. Accessed January 11, 2018.

16. Taylor, P. Bavarian Nordic tanks after Bristol-Myers-partnered vaccine flunks phase 3 prostate cancer trial. *Fierce Biotech.* September 15, 2017. https://www.fiercebiotech.com/biotech/bavarian-nordic-tanks-after-bristol-myers-part nered-vaccine-flunks-phase-3-prostate-cancer. Accessed August 2, 2019.

17. Clarke T. FDA aims to approve more drugs based on early clinical data. Health News. November 30, 2017. https://www.reuters.com/article/us-fda-hearing -testimony/fda-aims-to-approve-more-drugs-based-on-early-clinical-data-idUSKB N1DU2DS. Accessed July 28, 2019.

18. Tap W, Jones R, Van Tine B, Chmielowski B. et al. Olaratumab and doxorubicin versus doxorubicin alone for treatment of soft-tissue sarcoma: an open-label phase 1b and randomised phase 2 trial. *Lancet.* 2016;388(10043): P488–497. https://www.thelancet.com/journals/lancet/article/PIIS0140-6736(16) 30587-6/fulltext. Accessed July 28, 2019.

19. Olaratumab for STS disappoints in phase III. Cancer News. AACR. http:// cancerdiscovery.aacrjournals.org/content/early/2019/01/28/2159-8290.CD-NB 2019-011. Accessed July 28, 2019.

20. Ingram I. "Unprecedented" survival benefit vanishes in confirmatory can-cer trial—over $500 million in sales for drug with possibly no benefit. MedPage Today. June 3, 2019. https://www.medpagetoday.com/meetingcoverage/asco/80217. Accessed July 28, 2019.

21. Park JW, Finn RS, Kim JS, et al. Phase II, open-label study of brivanib as first-line therapy in patients with advanced hepatocellular carcinoma. *Clin Cancer Res.* 2011;17(7):1973–1983.

22. Llovet JM, Ricci S, Mazzaferro V, et al. Sorafenib in advanced hepato-cellular carcinoma. *New Engl J Med.* 2008;359(4):378–390.

23. Johnson PJ, Qin S, Park JW, et al. Brivanib versus sorafenib as first-line therapy in patients with unresectable, advanced hepatocellular carcinoma: results from the randomized phase III BRISK-FL study. *J Clin Oncol.* 2013;31(28):3517–3524.

24. Bristol-Myers Squibb. Comparison of brivanib and best supportive care (BSC) with placebo and BSC for treatment of liver cancer in Asian patients who have failed sorafenib treatment (BRISK-APS). Available from: https://clinicaltrials .gov/ct2/show/NCT01108705. NLM identifier: NCT01108705. Last update Oc-tober 12, 2015. Accessed August 2, 2019.

25. Kudo M, Han G, Finn RS, et al. Brivanib as adjuvant therapy to transarte-rial chemoembolization in patients with hepatocellular carcinoma: a randomized phase III trial. *Hepatology (Baltimore, Md).* 2014;60(5):1697–1707.

26. Ning YM, Suzman D, Maher VE, et al. FDA Approval summary: ate-zolizumab for the treatment of patients with progressive advanced urothelial carcinoma after platinum-containing chemotherapy. *Oncologist.* 2017;22(6): 743–749.

27. Roche provides update on phase III study of TECENTRIQ® (atezolizumab) in people with previously treated advanced bladder cancer [press release]. https:// www.roche.com/media/releases/med-cor-2017-05-10.htm. Roche, May 10, 2017.

28. FDA grants accelerated approval to pembrolizumab for advanced gastric cancer. 2017; September 22, 2017; https://www.fda.gov/Drugs/InformationOn Drugs/ApprovedDrugs/ucm577093.htm. Accessed January 11, 2018.

29. Broderick JM. Pembrolizumab Misses endpoints in phase III gastric cancer trial. *News* 2017; http://www.onclive.com/web-exclusives/pembrolizumab-misses -endpoints-in-phase-iii-gastric-cancer-trial. Accessed January 11, 2018.

30. Chen L, Li T, Fang F, Zhang Y, Faramand A. Tight glycemic control in critically ill pediatric patients: a systematic review and meta-analysis. *Crit Care.* 2018;22:57.

31. Antonia SJ, López-Martin JA, Bendell J, et al. Nivolumab alone and nivolumab plus ipilimumab in recurrent small-cell lung cancer (CheckMate 032): a multicentre, open-label, phase 1/2 trial. *Lancet Oncol.* 2016;17(7):883–895.

32. Bristol-Myers Squibb announces phase 3 CheckMate-331 study does not meet primary endpoint of overall survival with Opdivo versus chemotherapy in patients with previously treated relapsed small cell lung cancer [press release]. https://news.bms.com/press-release/corporatefinancial-news/bristol-myers-squibb -announces-phase-3-checkmate-498-study-did. Bristol-Myers Squibb, October 12, 2018.

33. Gill J, Prasad V. A reality check of the accelerated approval of immune-checkpoint inhibitors. *Nat Rev Clin Oncol.* (2019).

34. Prasad V. The withdrawal of drugs for commercial reasons: the incomplete story of tositumomab. *JAMA Intern Med.* 2014 Dec;174(12):1887–88. https:// www.ncbi.nlm.nih.gov/pubmed/25383420. Accessed July 28, 2019.

35. Barclay L. FDA approves cetuximab for advanced colorectal cancer: an expert interview with Howard Hochster, MD. 2004. https://www.medscape.com /viewarticle/469463. Accessed January 11, 2018.

36. Jonker DJ, O'Callaghan CJ, Karapetis CS, et al. Cetuximab for the treatment of colorectal cancer. *New Engl J Med.* 2007;357(20):2040–2048.

37. Burotto M, Prasad V, Fojo T. Non-inferiority trials: why oncologists must remain wary. *Lancet Oncol.* 2015;16(4):364–366.

38. Lang I, Brodowicz T, Ryvo L, et al. Bevacizumab plus paclitaxel versus bevacizumab plus capecitabine as first-line treatment for HER2-negative metastatic breast cancer: interim efficacy results of the randomised, open-label, non-inferiority, phase 3 TURANDOT trial. *Lancet Oncol.* 2013;14(2):125–133.

39. Aberegg S, Hersh A, Samore M. Empirical consequences of current recommendations for the design and interpretation of noninferiority trials. *J Gen Intern Med.* 2018 January;33(1):88–96. https://www.ncbi.nlm.nih.gov/pmc/articles /PMC5756156/. Accessed August 9, 2019.

40. Flacco ME, Manzoli L, Boccia S, et al. Head-to-head randomized trials are mostly industry sponsored and almost always favor the industry sponsor. *J Clin Epidemiol.* 2015;68(7):811–820.

41. Kudo M, Finn RS, Qin S, et al. Lenvatinib versus sorafenib in first-line treatment of patients with unresectable hepatocellular carcinoma: a randomised phase 3 non-inferiority trial. *Lancet.* 2018;391(10126):1163–1173.

42. Motzer RJ, Hutson TE, Cella D, et al. Pazopanib versus sunitinib in metastatic renal-cell carcinoma. *New Engl J Med.* 2013;369(8):722–731.

43. San Miguel JF, Schlag R, Khuageva NK, et al. Bortezomib plus melphalan

and prednisone for initial treatment of multiple myeloma. *New Engl J Med.* 2008; 359(9):906–917.

44. Coiffier B, Lepage E, Brière J, et al. CHOP chemotherapy plus rituximab compared with CHOP alone in elderly patients with diffuse large-B-cell lymphoma. *New Engl J Med.* 2002;346(4):235–242.

45. Buckner JC, Shaw EG, Pugh SL, et al. Radiation plus procarbazine, CCNU, and vincristine in low-grade glioma. *New Engl J Med.* 2016;374(14):1344–1355.

Chapter 12. Global Oncology

1. Farmer P, Frenk J, Knaul FM, et al. Expansion of cancer care and control in countries of low and middle income: a call to action. *Lancet.* 2010;376(9747): 1186–1193.

2. Goldstein DA, Clark J, Tu Y, et al. A global comparison of the cost of patented cancer drugs in relation to global differences in wealth. *Oncotarget.* 2017;8(42):71548–71555.

3. Prasad V, Mailankody S. The UK cancer drugs fund experiment and the US cancer drug cost problem. *Mayo Clin Proc.* 91(6):707–712.

4. New 50 million pound cancer fund already intellectually bankrupt. *Lancet.* 2010;376(9739):389.

5. The Cancer Drugs Fund is a costly mistake. *Opinon FT View* 2014; https://www.ft.com/content/616c851a-8211-11e4-b9d0-00144feabdco. Accessed February 2, 2018.

6. Le Fanu J. Health Secretary Jeremy Hunt and a "creative" use of statistics. *Health Advice* 2014; http://www.telegraph.co.uk/lifestyle/wellbeing/healthadvice /11290455/Health-Secretary-Jeremy-Hunt-and-a-creative-use-of-statistics.html. Accessed February 2, 2018.

7. Prasad V, Kumar H, Mailankody S. Ethics of clinical trials in low-resource settings: lessons from recent trials in cancer medicine. *Journal of Global Oncology.* 2016;2(1):1–3.

8. Davies W. India has most cervical cancer deaths. *Wall Street Journal.* May 10, 2013.

9. Shastri SS, Mittra I, Mishra GA, et al. Effect of VIA screening by primary health workers: randomized controlled study in Mumbai, India. *JNCI: J Natl Cancer I* 2014;106(3):dju009. doi:10.1093/jnci/dju009.

10. Ortega B, Ethical questions linger in cervical-cancer study. *USA Today.* August 31, 2013. http://www.usatoday.com/story/news/nation/2013/08/31/ethical -questions-linger-in-cervical-cancer-study/2751705.

11. Slamon DJ, Leyland-Jones B, Shak S, et al. Use of chemotherapy plus a monoclonal antibody against HER2 for metastatic breast cancer that overexpresses HER2. *New Engl J Med.* 2001;344(11):783–792.

12. Jahanzeb M. Continuing trastuzumab beyond progression. *J Clin Oncol.* 2009;27(12):1935–1937.

13. Mok TS, Wu Y-I., Thongprasert S, et al. Gefitinib or carboplatin-paclitaxel in pulmonary adenocarcinoma. *New Engl J Med.* 2009;361(10):947–957.

14. Sequist LV, Yang JC, Yamamoto N, et al. Phase III study of afatinib or cisplatin plus pemetrexed in patients with metastatic lung adenocarcinoma with EGFR mutations. *J Clin Oncol.* 2013;31(27):3327–3334.

15. Wu YL, Zhou C, Hu CP, et al. Afatinib versus cisplatin plus gemcitabine for first-line treatment of Asian patients with advanced non-small-cell lung cancer harbouring EGFR mutations (LUX-Lung 6): an open-label, randomised phase 3 trial. *Lancet Oncol.* 2014;15(2):213–222.

16. Flanigan RC, Salmon SE, Blumenstein BA, et al. Nephrectomy followed by Interferon Alfa-2b compared with Interferon Alfa-2b alone for metastatic renal-cell cancer. *New Engl J Med.* 2001;345(23):1655–1659.

17. Méjean A, Ravaud A, Thezenas S, et al. Sunitinib alone or after nephrectomy in metastatic renal-cell carcinoma. *New Engl J Med.* 2018;379(5):417–427.

18. Khan SA, Stewart AK, Morrow M. Does aggressive local therapy improve survival in metastatic breast cancer? *Surgery.* 2002;132(4):620–626; discussion 626–627.

19. Babiera GV, Rao R, Feng L, et al. Effect of primary tumor extirpation in breast cancer patients who present with stage IV disease and an intact primary tumor. *Ann Surg Oncol.* 2006;13(6):776–782.

20. Rapiti E, Verkooijen HM, Vlastos G, et al. Complete excision of primary breast tumor improves survival of patients with metastatic breast cancer at diagnosis. *J Clin Oncol.* 2006;24(18):2743–2749.

21. Gnerlich J, Jeffe DB, Deshpande AD, Beers C, Zander C, Margenthaler JA. Surgical removal of the primary tumor increases overall survival in patients with metastatic breast cancer: analysis of the 1988–2003 SEER data. *Ann Surg Oncol.* 2007;14(8):2187–2194.

22. Fields RC, Jeffe DB, Trinkaus K, et al. Surgical resection of the primary tumor is associated with increased long-term survival in patients with stage IV breast cancer after controlling for site of metastasis. *Ann Surg Oncol.* 2007;14(12): 3345–3351.

23. Blanchard DK, Shetty PB, Hilsenbeck SG, Elledge RM. Association of surgery with improved survival in stage IV breast cancer patients. *Ann Surg.* 2008; 247(5):732–738.

24. Rao R, Feng L, Kuerer HM, et al. Timing of surgical intervention for the intact primary in stage IV breast cancer patients. *Ann Surg Oncol.* 2008;15(6): 1696–1702.

25. Petrelli F, Barni S. Surgery of primary tumors in stage IV breast cancer: an updated meta-analysis of published studies with meta-regression. *Med Oncol* (Northwood, London, England). 2012;29(5):3282–3290.

26. Badwe R, Hawaldar R, Nair N, et al. Locoregional treatment versus no treatment of the primary tumour in metastatic breast cancer: an open-label randomised controlled trial. *Lancet Oncol.* 16(13):1380–1388.

27. Noronha V, Joshi A, Patil VM, et al. Once-a-week versus once-every-3-weeks cisplatin chemoradiation for locally advanced head and neck cancer: a phase III randomized noninferiority trial. *J Clin Oncol.* 2017:Jco2017749457.

Chapter 13. How Should Cancer Drug Development Proceed?

1. Ivanova A, Paul B, Marchenko O, Song G, Patel N, Moschos SJ. Nine-year change in statistical design, profile, and success rates of phase II oncology trials. *J Biopharm Stat.* 2016;26(1):141–149.

2. Djulbegovic B, Hozo I, Ioannidis JP. Improving the drug development process: more not less randomized trials. *JAMA.* 2014;311(4):355–356.

3. Prasad V, McCabe C, Mailankody S. Low-value approvals and high prices might incentivize ineffective drug development. *Nat Rev Clin Oncol.* 2018;15(7): 399–400.

4. Kiu T-T, Ilbawi, A Hill S. Comparison of sales income and research and development costs for FDA-approved cancer drugs sold by originator drug companies. *JAMA Netw Open.* 2019;2(1):e186875. https://jamanetwork.com /journals/jamanetworkopen/fullarticle/2720075

5. Martinez J. Driving drug innovation and market access: part 1—clinical trial cost breakdown. *News&Events Blog* 2016; https://www.centerpointclinicalservices .com/blog-posts/driving-drive-drug-innovation-and-market-access-part-1-clinical -trial-cost-breakdown/. Accessed January 2, 2018.

6. Zhu AX, Kudo M, Assenat E, et al. Effect of everolimus on survival in advanced hepatocellular carcinoma after failure of sorafenib: the EVOLVE-1 randomized clinical trial. *JAMA.* 2014;312(1):57–67.

7. Gbolahan OB, Schacht MA, Beckley EW, LaRoche TP, O'Neil BH, Pyko M. Locoregional and systemic therapy for hepatocellular carcinoma. *J Gastrointest Oncol.* 2017;8(2):215–228.

8. Gyawali B, Addeo A. Negative phase 3 randomized controlled trials: why cancer drugs fail the last barrier? *Intl J Cancer.* 2018;143(8):2079–2081.

9. Sacher AG, Le LW, Leighl NB. Shifting patterns in the interpretation of phase III clinical trial outcomes in advanced non-small-cell lung cancer: the bar is dropping. *J Clin Oncol.* 2014;32(14):1407–1411.

10. Del Paggio JC, Azariah B, Sullivan R, et al. Do contemporary randomized controlled trials meet ESMO thresholds for meaningful clinical benefit? *Ann Oncol.* 2017;28(1):157–162.

11. Gyawali B, Prasad V. Drugs that lack single-agent activity: are they worth pursuing in combination? *Nat Rev Clin Oncol.* 2017;14:193.

12. Chvetzoff Gl, Tannock IF. Placebo effects in oncology. *JNCI: J Natl Cancer I.* 2003;95(1):19–29.

13. Vaduganathan M, Prasad V. Modern drug development: which patients should come first? *JAMA.* 2014;312.

14. Chen E, Joshi S, Tran A, et al. Estimation of study time reduction using surrogate end points rather than overall survival in oncology clinical trials. *JAMA Intern Med.* 2019;179(5):642–647. https://jamanetwork.com/journals/jamainternal medicine/fullarticle/2729389.

15. Korn EL, Freidlin B. Adaptive clinical trials: advantages and disadvantages of various adaptive design elements. *JNCI: J Natl Cancer I.* 2017;109(6) doi:10 .1093/jnci/djx013.

16. Statler A, Radivoyevitch T, Siebenaller C, et al. Eligibility criteria are not associated with expected or observed adverse events in randomized controlled trials (RCTs) of hematologic malignancies. *Blood.* 2015;126(23): 635.

17. Dreicer JJ, Mailankody S, Fahkrejahani F, Prasad V. Clinically meaningful benefit: real world use compared against the American and European guidelines. *Blood Cancer J.* 2017;7(12):645.

18. Prasad V, Cifu A, Ioannidis JA. Reversals of established medical practices: evidence to abandon ship. *JAMA*. 2012;307(1):37–38.

19. Prasad V. Translation failure and medical reversal: Two sides to the same coin. *Eur J Cancer*. 2016;52:197–200.

20. Prasad V, Oseran A. Do we need randomised trials for rare cancers? *Eur J Cancer*. 51(11):1355–1357.

21. Fassnacht M, Terzolo M, Allolio B, et al. Combination chemotherapy in advanced adrenocortical carcinoma. *New Engl J Med*. 2012;366(23):2189–2197.

22. ASCO. Adrenal gland tumor: statistics. *Adrenal Gland Tumor* 2016; https://www.cancer.net/cancer-types/adrenal-gland-tumor/statistics. Accessed January 2, 2018.

23. Gaddipati H, Liu K, Pariser A, Pazdur R. Rare cancer trial design: lessons from FDA approvals. *Clin Cancer Res*. 2012;18(19):5172–5178.

Chapter 14. What Can Three Federal Agencies Do Tomorrow?

1. Misconceptions about FDA: 1. We don't set standards of care. 2. We don't have anything to do w drug pricing. 3. We don't have comparative efficacy standard. Drugs don't have to be better than avail therapy—Pazdur #SABCS17. Twitter 2017. https://twitter.com/FDAOncology/status/938422008534175745. Accessed February 13, 2018.

2. Tao D, Prasad V. Choice of control group in randomised trials of cancer medicine: are we testing trivialities? *Lancet Oncol*. 2018;19:1150–1152.

3. IMBRUVICA® (ibrutinib) [package insert]. Sunnyvale, CA: Pharmacyclics, LLC; US Food and Drug Administration, 2013. https://www.accessdata.fda.gov/drugsatfda_docs/label/2017/205552s016lbl.pdf. Accessed February 13, 2018.

4. FDA Approves Ibrutinib as Initial CLL Treatment. Medscape 2016. https://www.medscape.com/viewarticle/859911. Accessed February 13, 2018.

5. Burger JA, Tedeschi A, Barr PM, et al. Ibrutinib as Initial Therapy for Patients with Chronic Lymphocytic Leukemia. *New Engl J Med*. 2015;373:2425–2437.

6. Robert C, Long GV, Brady B, et al. Nivolumab in previously untreated melanoma without BRAF mutation. *New Engl J Med*. 2015;372:320–330.

7. OPDIVO (nivolumab) [package insert]. Princeton, NJ: Bristol-Myers Squibb Company; US Food and Drug Administration, 2014. https://www.accessdata.fda.gov/drugsatfda_docs/label/2018/125554s058lbl.pdf. Accessed February 13, 2018.

8. Hilal T, Sonbol M, Prasad V. Analysis of control arm quality in randomized clinical trials leading to anticancer drug approval by the US Food and Drug Administration. *JAMA Oncol*. 2019;5(6):887–892. https://jamanetwork.com/journals/jamaoncology/article-abstract/2732506.

9. FDA approves bortezomib regimen for untreated MCL. OncLive, 2014. http://www.onclive.com/web-exclusives/fda-approves-bortezomib-for-untreated-mantle-cell-lymphoma. Accessed February 13, 2018.

10. Robak T, Huang H, Jin J, et al. Bortezomib-based therapy for newly diagnosed mantle-cell lymphoma. *New Engl J Med*. 2015;372:944–953.

11. Robak T, Huang H, Jin J, et al. Supplement to: Robak T, Huang H, Jin J, et al. Bortezomib-based therapy for newly diagnosed mantle cell lymphoma. *New Engl J Med*. 2015;372(10):944–953.

12. Durkee BY, Qian Y, Pollom EL, et al. Cost-effectiveness of pertuzumab in human epidermal growth factor receptor 2–positive metastatic breast cancer. *J Clin Oncol.* 2016;34:902–909.

13. Swain SM, Kim SB, Cortés J, Ro J, Semiglazov V, Campone M. Pertuzumab, trastuzumab, and docetaxel for HER2-positive metastatic breast cancer (CLEOPATRA study): overall survival results from a randomised, double-blind, placebo-controlled, phase 3 study. *Lancet Oncol.* 2013;14.

14. Gyawali B, Prasad V. Health policy: Me-too drugs with limited benefits—the tale of regorafenib for HCC. *Nat Rev Clin Oncol.* 2017;14:653–654.

15. Bruix J, Qin S, Merle P, et al. Regorafenib for patients with hepatocellular carcinoma who progressed on sorafenib treatment (RESORCE): a randomised, double-blind, placebo-controlled, phase 3 trial. *Lancet* 2017;389:56–66.

16. Sanoff HK, Chang Y, Lund JL, O'Neil BH, Dusetzina SB. Sorafenib effectiveness in advanced hepatocellular carcinoma. *Oncologist.* 2016;21:1113–1120.

17. Lee IC, et al. Determinants of survival after sorafenib failure in patients with BCLC-C hepatocellular carcinoma in real-world practice. *Medicine* (Baltimore) 94;e688 (2015).

18. Chen E, Raghunathan V, Prasad V. An overview of cancer drugs approved by the US Food and Drug Administration based on the surrogate end point of response rate. *JAMA Intern Med.* 2019;179(7):915–921. https://www.ncbi.nlm.nih.gov/pubmed/31135822.

19. Gyawali B, Hey SP, Kesselheim AS. Assessment of the Clinical Benefit of Cancer Drugs Receiving Accelerated Approval. *JAMA Intern Med.* 2019;179(7): 906–913. https://www.ncbi.nlm.nih.gov/pubmed/31135808.

20. Bekelman JE, Joffe S. Three steps toward a more sustainable path for targeted cancer drugs. *JAMA.* 2018;319:2167–2168.

21. Downing NS, Zhang AD, Ross JS. Regulatory review of new therapeutic agents—FDA versus EMA, 2011–2015. *New Engl J Med.* 2017;376:1386–1387.

22. Wagner J, Marquart J, Ruby J, et al. Frequency and level of evidence used in recommendations by the National Comprehensive Cancer Network guidelines beyond approvals of the US Food and Drug Administration: retrospective observational study. *BMJ.* 2018;360.

23. Prasad V. The folly of big science awards. *New York Times.* October 2, 2015.

24. Levitt M, Levitt JM. Future of fundamental discovery in US biomedical research. *P Nl A Sci.* 2017;114:6498.

25. Gould J. Should we patch the leaky PhD pipeline? *Nature Jobs Blog;* http://blogs.nature.com/naturejobs/2014/09/02/should-we-patch-the-leaky-pipeline/. 2014.

26. Nicholson JM, Ioannidis JPA. Conform and be funded. *Nature.* 2012;492:34.

27. Kaiser J. Critics challenge NIH finding that bigger labs aren't necessarily better. *Science.* June 7, 2017.

28. Ioannidis JPA. Fund people not projects. *Nature.* 2011;477:529.

Chapter 15. What Can People with Cancer Do?

1. Kutner JS, Blatchford PJ, Taylor DH, Jr., et al. Safety and benefit of discontinuing statin therapy in the setting of advanced, life-limiting illness: a randomized clinical trial. *JAMA Intern Med.* 2015;175(5):691–700.

2. Mody P, Nguyen OK. Selecting the optimal design for drug discontinuation trials in a setting of advanced, life-limiting illness. *JAMA Intern Med.* 2015; 175(10):1725.

3. US Food & Drug Administration. FDA voices: perspectives from FDA experts. https://www.fda.gov/newsevents/newsroom/fdavoices/default.htm. Accessed August 2, 2019.

Chapter 16. What Can Students, Residents, and Fellows Do?

1. Ioannidis JP. Evidence-based medicine has been hijacked: a report to David Sackett. *Journal of Clinical Epidemiology.* 2016;73:82–86.

Epilogue

1. Prasad V, Rajkumar SV. Conflict of interest in academic oncology: moving beyond the blame game and forging a path forward. *Blood Cancer Journal.* 2016;6(11):e489.

2. Gyawali B, Kesselheim AS. US Food and Drug Administration approval of new drugs based on noninferiority trials in oncology: a dangerous precedent? US Food and Drug Administration Approval of New Drugs Based on Noninferiority Trials in Oncology. 2019.

3. Prasad V. Non-inferiority trials in medicine: practice changing or a self-fulfilling prophecy? *J Gen Intern Med.* 2018;33(1):3–5.

4. Prasad V, Massey PR, Fojo T. Oral anticancer drugs: how limited dosing options and dose reductions may affect outcomes in comparative trials and efficacy in patients. *Journal of Clinical Oncology.* 2014;32(15):1620–1629.

5. Tao D, Prasad V. Choice of control group in randomised trials of cancer medicine: are we testing trivialities? *Lancet Oncology.* 2018;19(9):1150–1152.

6. Prasad V, De Jesus K, Mailankody S. The high price of anticancer drugs: origins, implications, barriers, solutions. *Nature Reviews Clinical oncology.* 2017;14(6):381–390.

7. NHE Fact Sheet. Centers for Medicare & Medicaid Services National Health Expenditure Data Web site. https://www.cms.gov/research-statistics-data-and -systems/statistics-trends-and-reports/nationalhealthexpenddata/nhe-fact-sheet .html. Published 2019. Updated April 4. Accessed May 14, 2019.

8. Dunn A. Drugmakers say R&D spending hit record in 2017. Biopharma Dive https://www.biopharmadive.com/news/phrma-research-development-spending -industry-report/529943/. Published 2018. Updated August 13. Accessed May 14, 2019.

9. Health NIH. Budget. https://www.nih.gov/about-nih/what-we-do/budget #note. Published 2019. Accessed May 14, 2019.

10. CMS finalizes coverage of Next Generation Sequencing tests, ensuring enhanced access for cancer patients [press release]. CMS.gov. March 16, 2018.

11. Prasad V. Why the US Centers for Medicare and Medicaid Services (CMS) should have required a randomized trial of Foundation Medicine (F1CDx) before paying for it. *Annals of Oncology.* 2018;29(2):298–300.

12. Sicklick JK, Kato S, Okamura R, et al. Molecular profiling of cancer patients enables personalized combination therapy: the I-PREDICT study. *Nature Medicine.* 2019;25(5):744–750.

13. Sicklick JK, Leyland-Jones B, Kato S, et al. Personalized, molecularly matched combination therapies for treatment-na. *Journal of Clinical Oncology.* 2017;35(15_suppl):2512–2512.

14. CMS finalizes coverage of Next Generation Sequencing tests, ensuring enhanced access for cancer patients [press release]. CMS.gov. March 16, 2018.

15. Contopoulos-Ioannidis DG, Ntzani E, Ioannidis JP. Translation of highly promising basic science research into clinical applications. *Am J Med.* 2003;114(6): 477–484.

16. Bella T. A Texas scientist was called "foolish" for arguing the immune system could fight cancer. Then he won the Nobel Prize. *Washington Post.* March 25, 2019.

17. Marquart J, Chen EY, Prasad V. Estimation of the percentage of US patients with cancer who benefit from genome-driven oncology. *JAMA Oncology.* 2018; 4(8):1093–1098.

18. Joyner MJ, Paneth N, Ioannidis JP. What happens when underperforming big ideas in research become entrenched? *JAMA.* 2016;316(13):1355–1356.

19. Fang FC, Bowen A, Casadevall A. NIH peer review percentile scores are poorly predictive of grant productivity. *eLife.* 2016;5:e13323.

20. Mayo NE, Brophy J, Goldberg MS, et al. Peering at peer review revealed high degree of chance associated with funding of grant applications. *J Clin Epidemiol.* 2006;59(8):842–848.

21. Marsh HW, Jayasinghe UW, Bond NW. Improving the peer-review process for grant applications: reliability, validity, bias, and generalizability. *American Psychologist.* 2008;63(3):160–168.

22. Pagano M. American Idol and NIH grant review. *Cell.* 2006;126(4):637–638.

23. Bollen J, Crandall D, Junk D, Ding Y, Börner K. From funding agencies to scientific agency: collective allocation of science funding as an alternative to peer review. *EMBO Reports.* 2014;15(2):131–133.

24. Ioannidis JPA. Fund people not projects. *Nature.* 2011;477:529.

25. Fang FC, Casadevall A. Research funding: the case for a modified lottery. *mBio.* 2016;7(2):e00422–00416.

26. Tao DL, Gay ND, Prasad V. Statistical significance of bevacizumab trials when considering the portfolio of all studies. *Journal of Clinical Oncology.* 2018;36(15_suppl):6551–6551.

Page numbers in *italics* indicate figures and tables.

Food and Drug Administration (*cont.*)
86; post-protocol therapy and, 203,
205, 207–9; rare diseases and,
198–99; regular approval from, 11,
37–38, 40; requirements for approval
of, 186, 187; revolving door between
biopharmaceutical companies and,
87–88, 102; size of benefit and, 214;
surrogate endpoints and, 28, 37–39,
213–14; trials in developing world
and, 170–71. *See also* accelerated
approval by FDA
Foundation Medicine, 107, 243
Fugh-Berman, A., 96
funding of research: by government,
63, 160; grants, 219; by industry, 56,
102, 133–34; inefficiency of, 244,
245; non-inferiority trials and,
162–63; recommendations for, 218

Gale, Robert Peter, 106
"game changer," use of term, 68–69
gefitinib, 174
gemcitabine, 138–39
gemtuzumab ozogamicin, 29
genetic mutations and drug benefit,
159–60
genetic sequencing, 109, 112
GENIE, 107
Gill, Jennifer, 158, 161
global oncology: clinical trials in
developing world, 170–79; cost of
drugs and, 167; definition of, 166
goal of treatment, 137, 222
Goldstein, Dan, 167
Gottlieb, Scott, 73, 155
government: funding by, 61–62, 63,
194; as maximizing welfare of
people, 167–68, 170; revolving door
between industry and, 87–88, 102
Grady, Christine, 131
Guardiant, 107
guidelines specific to each cancer, 80
Gyawali, Bishal, 33, 187, 188

halting trials for futility, 154–55
Hanley, J. A., 25
Haslam, Alyson, 161
hazard ratio, 70–71, 162

health care, money spent on, 17
HER2-directed drugs, 36, 173–74, 183,
209
high blood pressure, treatment of,
17–18
Hilal, Talal, 206
historically controlled studies, 60,
126–28
Howard, D., 58
hyping of novel therapies: autologous
stem cell transplant, 3–4; "cure" as,
71–72; dangers of, 6; definition of,
67; "inflection point," use of term,
72–73; in lay press, 68–71; palbociclib, 67–68; by patients in news
stories, 76–77; in press releases,
74–75; in professional meetings,
75–76

ibrutinib, 203–5, 204
imatinib, 11–12, 15, 26, 49, 68
immunotherapy drugs, 51
IMPACT-2 trial, 111
improvement, striving for, 235
independence, in cancer policy, 239–41
India, cancer trials in, 172–73, 177–78,
178, 180
indolent biology, selecting for, 60–61
industry. *See* biopharmaceutical
companies
"inflection point," use of term, 72–73
information and literature, keeping up
with, 231–34
informative censoring, 44–45
iniparib, 153–54
intention to treat principle, 43
interventions in randomized controlled
trials, 124–25
investigations to work up diagnoses,
146–47
Ioannidis, John, 197, 219
Iodine 131-tositumomab, 159, 213
irinotecan, 118, 138
IV medication, payments for administration of, 102

Joffe, Steven, 214
Joshi, Sunil, 34
June, Carl, 62

quality adjusted life-year (QALY),
16–17
quality of life, surrogate endpoints as
predictors of, 33

Rajkumar, Vincent, 102
randomized controlled trials (RCTs):
of autologous stem cell transplant,
4; benefits of, 125; of bevacizumab,
123–24, 125–26; clinically meaningful benefits reported by, 188; control
groups for, 130, 195–96, 203, 204–7;
cost of, 185; crossover in, 128–33;
following observational studies,
122–23; historically controlled
studies compared with, 127–28;
importance of, 5; multiplicity and,
125, 134–35; of precision oncology,
111–13, *113*; prerequisites for, 124;
of ProMACE-cytaBOM, 127; for
rare diseases, 197–99; sample size
and, 133–34, 153–56, 187–88; use
of drugs based on, 138–39
rare diseases, randomized controlled
trials for, 197–99
real-world data, 229
RECIST (Response Evaluation Criteria
in Solid Tumors), 25, 27–28, 140
recurrence, 33
refractory tumors, 51
registration studies, 170–71
regorafenib, 17, 192, 211, 211–12
regression to mean, 155–56
regulatory system, successful, metric of,
165
relapsed tumors, 51
relative risk, 123n
relevance, in cancer policy, 241–42
Relman, Arnold, 98–99
research: acronyms for, 123n; financial
conflicts of interest in, 19; separating
health care and, 242–43. *See also*
funding of research; randomized
controlled trials; trials in drug
development
research and development (R&D): costs
of drugs in, 19–21, 54–55, 185; incentives for, 183–84, 185–87. *See also*
trials in drug development

researchers, as scientists, 117
research payments to doctors, 79
RESONATE-2 trial, 203–5, *204*
Response Oncology, 4
response rate, 213. *See also* tumor
shrinkage
Rini, B. I., 145
rituximab, 57, 163–64
rociletinib, 25–26
rosiglitazone, 96
Russell, M. H., 72

Sacher, Adrian, 187
sample size in randomized controlled
trials, 133–34, 153–56, 187–88
scientists, types of, 117
screening tests: CA-125, 149–50, *151*,
152–53; for cervical cancer, 172–73
second-line therapy, 137
selection bias, 43, 192
selumetinib, 153
sequencing tumors, 107–8, 243
sequential use of drugs, 142, 144
SHARP trial, 211
SHIVA trial, 111
Shkreli, Martin, 52
Silver, Sheldon, 92–93, *93*
single agent activity, as prerequisite for
drug development, 156, 188–89,
190–91
sipuleucel-T, 131–32
small molecules, 18, 51
Smith, Elaine, 2
social media, oncologists on, 81–84, *82*
Sonbol, Mohamad, 206
sorafenib: adjuvant setting and, 138;
comparison trials against, 157, 162,
187; control arms of trials of, 192;
R&D for, 55; regorafenib and, 211,
211–12; trial population for, 13–14
spinning negative studies, 73–74
stable disease, as response in trials, 156
standards of care for trials: best available US, 192, *193*, *194*; crossover
and, 130; in developing world,
170–71; FDA and, 203, 205, 207–9
statin drugs and terminal cancer,
227–29
Steinbrook, Robert, 100

stem cell transplant, autologous, 3–5

S-TRAC trial, 138

study designs: in drug development, 196–97, 214–16; historically controlled, 60, 126–28; selection of, 117–18; types of, 117; unethical, 173–74, 207. *See also* observational studies; randomized controlled trials

sunitinib, 138, 140–41, 162–63

surrogate endpoints: classes of, 24; in cost-effectiveness studies, 57; definition of, 23; evidence for, 33–34; FDA drug approvals and, 37–40, 213–14; hematologic response, 11–12; increase in use of, 28; measurement of, 23–24; as misleading, 29–30; as predictors of survival, 5, 30–33, *31, 32*; regulator comments on, 48–50; time savings from use of, 34–36, 193; time-to-event, 27–28; validation of, 38–39, 42. *See also* tumor shrinkage

surrogate threshold effects, 46–47

survival (living longer): drugs that improve, 21–22; response rate and, 27; surrogate endpoints as predictors of, 30–33, *31, 32*; trials that assess, 189, 192–93

survival post-protocol argument, 48, *49*

Tamiflu, 34

Tao, Derrick, 82, 203

targeted drugs, 51

Tata Medical Centre, Mumbai, 172, 177–79, *180*

Taub, Robert, 92–93

T-cells, 59

thought/key opinion leaders, 79–81

time-to-event endpoints, 27–28, 43–46, *46*

tisagenlecleucel, 43, 61–62

toxicity: in adjuvant settings, 137; of CAR-T, 59–60, 61; censoring patient data and, 44–45; of chemotherapy, 3; combining drugs, extending therapy, and, 142–43; crossover and, 132–33; of everolimus, 40; move to phase 2 trials and, 185; treating to progression and, 141

trainees, recommendations for, 231–37

transparency: in disclosure of funding sources, 103; in drug pricing, 55

trastuzumab, 173–74, 209

trials in drug development: advancing drugs and, 193–94, 207–9; aspirational, 163–64; cancer antigen 125, 149–50, *151, 152*–53; current system of, 184–88; design and conduct of, 196–97, 214–16; in developing world, 170–79; dose and schedule in, 194–95; non-inferiority trials, 161–63; overview of, 13–14, 164–65; paradigm of, 199–200; participation in, 225; patients in, 189, 192–93, 195, 210–12; patients lost to follow-up, 44; phases of, 184–85; power of, 196; single agent drugs in, 156, 188–89, *190–91*; strengthening structure of, 195–96; unethical, 207. *See also* nonconflicted trials agenda; randomized controlled trials; standards of care for trials; surrogate endpoints; tumor shrinkage; *specific named trials*

Tufts Center for the Study of Drug Development, 19

tumors, local treatment of, 175–78, *178*

tumor shrinkage (response rate): arbitrary threshold for, 24–25, 27, 36; drugs for, 21; measurement of, 25–27, 42–43; precision oncology and, 108–9; to qualify as game changer, 68; regulator comments on, 48–49; as surrogate endpoint, 3, 5, 24–25; trials in oncology and, 156–59

Turing Pharmaceuticals, 52–53

21st Century Cures Bill, 122

Twitter, oncologists on, 81–84, *82*

unidirectional crossover. *See* crossover

United Kingdom, cancer drug fund in, 167–70

United Nations Millennium Development Goals, 167

"unmet medical needs," 41, 184, 193

"unprecedented," use of term, 70–71

unpublished studies, 34

About the Author

Vinayak K. Prasad, MD, MPH, is an associate professor of medicine at the Oregon Health and Science University in Portland, Oregon. He is a practicing hematologist-oncologist and internal medicine physician. He completed his training at the National Cancer Institute and the National Institutes of Health in Bethesda, Maryland. Dr. Prasad's research focuses on oncology drugs, health policy, evidence-based medicine, bias, and medical reversal. Dr. Prasad is the author of more than 200 articles in academic journals. With Dr. Adam Cifu, he wrote *Ending Medical Reversal: Improving Outcomes, Saving Lives*. He is the host of the podcast *Plenary Session*. He is on Twitter @vprasadmdmph.